Healthy Beauty

Using Nature's Secrets
to Look Great and Feel Terrific

LETHA HADADY

Illustrated by
Letha Elizabeth Hadady

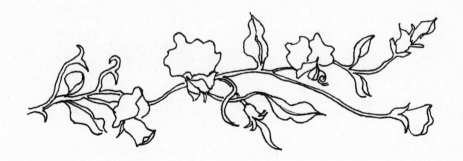

WILEY

John Wiley & Sons, Inc.

Published by John Wiley & Sons, Inc., Hoboken, New Jersey
Published simultaneously in Canada

39 illustrations by Letha Elizabeth Hadady; Used with permission.

For general information about our other products and services, please contact
our Customer Care Department within the United States at (800) 762-2974, outside
the United States at (317) 572-3993 or fax (317) 572-4002.

Wiley also publishes its books in a variety of electronic formats. Some content
that appears in print may not be available in electronic books.

Library of Congress Cataloging-in-Publication Data:

Hadady, Letha.
  Healthy beauty : using nature's secrets to look great and feel terrific / Letha Hadady.
      p. ; cm.
  Includes bibliographical references and index.
    ISBN 0-471-07534-5 (cloth)
  1. Beauty, Personal. 2. Women—Health and hygiene.
    [DNLM: 1. Beauty—Popular Works. 2. Health Behavior—Popular Works.
  3. Hygiene—Popular Works. QT 275 H125h 2003] I. Title.
    RA778 .H157 2003
    646.7'042—dc21

                                                                          2002014025

Printed in the United States of America
10 9 8 7 6 5 4 3 2 1

Also by Letha Hadady

Asian Health Secrets

Personal Renewal

In your heart you know you are beautiful and divine.

Holding a letter from Mother, I notice her fine longhand that glides with grace and confidence—an artist's hand. "A family of quails has roosted on the back patio," she writes. Early mornings the birds gather seeds that Mother has left for them in an earthen bowl. Sun-soaked, they gaze at the blue Sandia mountains. Last week a doe crossed the mesa and peeked over her fence. Black bear have reached the corridor that separates man and mountain. They are safe with Mother.

She embodies the loving spirit of benevolence and generosity that makes up the better part of civilization and nature—as ageless as the forest itself. Her house is filled with music. Her paintings of pansies, purple iris, and pink hollyhocks, of rolling streams meandering through shaded meadows, aspens turned glorious yellow, and wild geese watching expectantly in high blue grass mirror a unified ideal: Her art reveals the beauty she loves. In one painting, a mermaid reclines on an oyster shell, while holding a luminous, perfectly round pearl. A pearl has many layers made by years of ocean currents. It is an emblem of natural beauty, value, and purity. Mother and I dedicate this book to you and the pearl within.

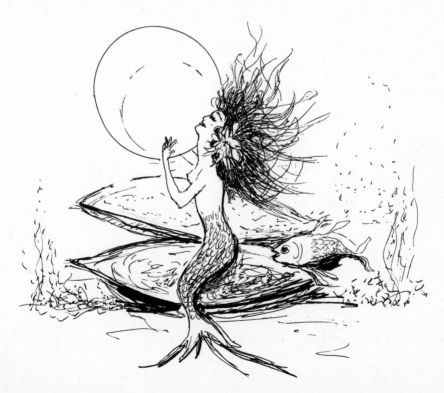

Contents

Part Four: Beauty Karma

Foreword

We have often heard the phrase, "Beauty is in the eye of the beholder." Beauty is an aggregate of qualities in a person or thing that gives pleasure to the senses . . . exalting the spirit!

Letha Hadady's *Healthy Beauty* is the first book of its kind. Descending from a long line of Hungarian beauties, Letha's skills have been honed pursuing natural beauty throughout the world. Letha marries three distinct cultures: Eastern European, Asian (Chinese and Ayurvedic medicine), and Western (the highly competitive cosmetic industry). *Healthy Beauty* is an international beauty recipe of tried and true home preparations blended with the most modern technologically advanced products on the market today.

Our mutual friend, Hollywood director Luke Yankee, introduced me to this high priestess of Asian medicine. Since our initial meeting we have been cast together listening, learning, and sharing in the knowledge of all things beautiful.

This book is truly a celebration of Beauty in all its diversity, reflecting with the author's individualized, energetic point of view that after all, "Beauty is more than skin deep."

—Clif de Raita,
National Director of Makeup,
Georgette Klinger, Inc.

Acknowledgments

I thank my beautiful sister Michelle for suggesting that I write this book. I am grateful for the fine artwork of my mother, Letha Elizabeth Hadady. Their love for me is an inspiration. I especially thank novelist, biographer, and historian Michael Foster for nurturing and protecting this book.

Special thanks go to super-stylists Gad Cohen, Clif deRaita at Georgette Klinger Inc., Virginia Fry at Avon Spa in New York, and Marietta Carter-Narcisse in Los Angeles. I also thank Astrid Bedrossian, Phyllis Apostole Turrin and Eileen Paley of Georgette Klinger, Niki Finkel at Origins, and Bob Macloud and Stephen Bychieurez, founders of Kiss My Face, Inc.

I thank my healing friends in New York, Susan and Frank from Lin Sisters Herb Shop, Dr. Lili Wu, Anwar Mahmud, Linda van Horn, Rita Ghiraldini, Dr. Rudolph Ballentine, Natalie Naigles, and R. D. Chin. Many thanks go to Lan and Keng Ong at Wing Hop Fung in Los Angeles. I have enjoyed working with Andrew Gaeddert, founder of Health Concerns; Michel Czehatowski, founder of East Earth Trade Winds; and distinguished author and healer, the late Dr. Bernard Jensen in California. For their expert advice and encouragement I thank my brother, Dr. Eric Hadady in Albuquerque; Dr. Andrew Weil in Arizona; Rita J. Miller-Huey in Florida; and Dr. Yves Requena in France.

From the fashion and entertainment world, I thank Cathy Curtain and Sharlot Batton. From Hollywood, I thank Michael York, producer Jacquie Jordan, director Luke B. Yankee, and Don Hill of Actor's Equity. A number of television personalities have helped me, especially Mary Mucci from Cablevision in New York and Kelly Dunn from NBC station WPTV in West Palm Beach. In New England, I thank my friends, Michelle Parent, Rob and Ruth Ann Barker, the Dartmouth College Library staff, and Ms. Antoinette Fern at the Harvard Theatre Collection. Many thanks to all who take the time to be beautiful.

Introduction:
Beauty Now and Forever

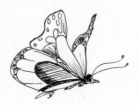

The shapely woman wrapped in a long coat over a T-shirt and jeans entered the empty dressing room. Without a word, the New York-born, Yale Drama School graduate took her place in the makeup chair. It was before coffee, the time of morning when every noise seemed loud. Marietta Carter-Narcisse tip-toed in and began hand-mixing the foundation she would apply to the beautiful face in the chair. The face was shut tight becoming Anna Mae Bullock, a sixteen-year-old waif from Nutbush, Tennessee.

Anna Mae and her sister were abandoned by their sharecropper parents in the segregated South. After her grandmother died, Anna Mae's education began in smoke-filled St. Louis R&B nightclubs. The girl had a son in her teens and swore that she would never leave him. She married a band leader who drank and then raped and beat her. The actress in the chair relaxed her face so that makeup could be applied.

Marietta glanced at her complexion. It was soft and flawless without using extra moisturizer. At times, Marietta recommends cleansing facial masks or a healthy diet of fresh fruits, vegetables, and lots of water. "The camera sees all imperfections," she would say. As she applied movie makeup, Marietta watched the transformation take place in the chair. The character on tour sang in smoke-filled joints while her husband took drugs. Suddenly it happened: Angela Bassett jumped up and *became* Tina Turner singing the refrain, "Rollin' on the river."

Angela Bassett was nominated for an Oscar and won both the Golden Globe and the NAACP Image Award for Outstanding Leading Actress for her portrayal of Tina Turner in the Touchstone Pictures 1993 movie, "What's Love Got to Do With It." Angela had never heard the Queen of Rock and Roll

1

sing before acting the part. The character was a result of the shared alchemy between actress, director, and makeup artist.

The ancient Egyptians recognized the power of makeup, whose daily application was considered a ritual offering to the gods. By recreating ourselves in front of a mirror daily, we join together what is inside and outside. When both blend smoothly, we feel whole, healthy, happy, and beautiful: We look in the mirror and see the person we want to see. Writing *Healthy Beauty* has forced me to reach deeper into myself and find what I had not recognized as beautiful. I eventually reclaimed the look of my eastern heritage.

I grew up speaking Hungarian in New Mexico. Back in the seventeenth century, the family name was changed from the Hungarian equivalent of "shoemaker" when an ancestor fought in the service of Leopold, the Holy Roman Emperor, to drive out the occupying Turks. The relative was knighted and granted the estate of a nobleman in the defeated Turkish army. Thus my quaint title as Hungarian countess.

My ancestors suffered from being Protestant in a Catholic country, and later from being labor organizers in a reactionary empire. They left Hungary for work in Chicago steel mills and later tried farming on the Canadian plains. The Hadadys came to New Mexico with the Manhattan Project that built the first atomic bomb. My father, who had worked on the Cyclotron at the University of Chicago, made miniature models of the Saturn rocket and the Sidewinder missile. A handsome man who liked to fish and hunt, he was exposed on the job to dangerous toxins and died young. My mother (and illustrator), despite being a lovely woman in every way, has never remarried.

Many Hungarians reflect the nation's origins on the steppes of Central Asia among a wandering Asiatic tribe. I have always supposed some subconscious memory of that time predisposed me to study traditional Asian medicines, and to apply my learning and experience to the subject of beauty. My quest has led me throughout the world and especially to the age-old traditions of China, India, and Tibet. For this book, I have consulted noted beauty gurus who work daily with models, actresses, as well as diplomatic and business professionals but also people who are familiar with their own ethnic herbal traditions.

Because all cultures use herbs, herbal traditions overlap. Tall, attractive Theresa Jackson, Assistant Vice President at The JP Morgan Chase Bank, originally from Jamaica, let me sample her Cerassie Tea (Momordica charantia), which she keeps in the office. "In Jamaica" she told me, "the tea is used to cleanse the entire body and reduce fat." I recognized the taste as bitter gourd used throughout Asia for reducing indigestion, blemishes, and diabetes. The tea is available at Asian markets and at internet sources listed in the Annotated Resource Guide. I am happy to share international beauty secrets with you. Reading this book, you can reach into your roots to create a unique beauty persona. Because natural beauty encompasses energy, vitality, sexual allure, and spiritual unfolding, the sky is the limit to your perfection.

This book takes inspiration from Lola Montez, a nineteenth century countess and herbalist, who wrote the first world-renowned bestseller on natural beauty. We both agree that the enemy of beauty is not age but illness, attitude, and lifestyle. This book can improve beauty skills in order to create your unique beauty persona. That requires observation and reflection from you. On 57th street near Carnegie Hall, I asked my friend Jacquie Jordan, a Los Angeles-based daytime television producer, "How are the New York and Los Angeles looks different?" We watched a woman with short gray hair, wearing a black wool cape, black leggings, and tall black boots cross the street. "That's very New York," she replied. "In L.A., you wear colors and open-toe shoes. The latest thing is pink sunglasses shaped like hearts. In L.A. you dress to be seen. In New York, you dress to remain anonymous." Do you dress to be seen or ignored? Too often, we dress without thinking: we deny our natural gifts. This book can help you express confidence and personal power.

A Beautiful, Healthy You

Beauty is an ensemble. Your walk, voice, clothes, and style add or detract from your appeal to others. Pleasing breath and body odor are essential and achievable with diet and herbs rather than a drug store deodorant. Any serious discordance can ruin the total effect. For that reason, I have treated as beauty issues health topics generally not addressed in beauty books. Beauty encompasses who you are and what you want in life.

Vitality is evident from good posture, glowing skin, bright eyes, thick, shiny hair, and smooth fingernails. Unfortunately, our lifestyle is often not healthy. Cathy Curtin, a vivacious Actor's Studio performer with Broadway, film, and television credits, created the role of Fran Richtken on "Guiding Light." Currently, she is portraying singer Janis Joplin at the Village Theater. The tough role demands daily smoking. Her flawless skin requires protection. Cooling moisture creams, cleansing diet, and herbs found in this book can help us all deal with secondary smoke and pollution.

Beauty is in danger now more than ever before. Because we are only as safe as our air, water, food, and lifestyle habits, beauty information that stresses enhanced immunity is vital. Most of us recognize that we live in a dangerous world where civilians are the target of choice. The real possibility of facing chemical poisons, killer germs, and even atomic radiation is reason for concern. *Healthy Beauty* is the first book to address these as issues affecting the appearance of men and women. Chapter 17, Beauty Survival Skills, admittedly only a beginning, combats the dangers with natural remedies. The materials and methods for creating well-being have existed for generations in Western and Asian natural medicines. We will apply them in order to build your beauty and immunity from the inside out.

I have spent years investigating the close connection between health and beauty with an extensive practice using the tools of traditional Chinese medicine—acupuncture, massage, and herbs. I have been impressed by the desire of people, regardless of their health issues, to remain attractive. Teaching on both coasts and writing a weekly column for the internet, I receive ever more questions on maintaining beauty despite serious illnesses, or the harsh effects of medical drugs. Fortunately, the nature of herbal remedies is: what makes you look good makes you feel good.

In *Healthy Beauty,* using simple diagnostic tools borrowed from traditional Chinese medicine, you will learn to recognize the best foods, herbs, and natural treatments to suit your needs. People in a hurry can look for "Quick Fix" sections in many chapters. Those who seek the deeper meaning of beauty, the development of a personal aesthetic or beauty persona, will enjoy the "Lola's Way" sections.

Natural Secrets

Traditional Asian beauty remedies are the products of an ancient science, originally formulated for the well-being of the household of the Emperor and Empress of China, Japan, or Thailand, or the royal courts of India. These secret remedies, used by mandarins and the middle-classes, have been relied on for centuries by tens of millions of people. Actively and successfully used today, traditional beauty products work on a deep level to purify the body of toxins that threaten vitality and appearance. For example, *ashitaba* root, used in Japanese cooking, clarifies the skin while reducing cholesterol. *Konnyaku* noodle is an excellent weight-loss food because it contains no calories. Both foods are easily available as standardized capsules from a Japanese-American manufacturer in Los Angeles.

Anywhere you will find Asians you will find unusual looking mushrooms. Polysaccharides found in Asian mushrooms provide immunity to illness as well as a potent source of absorbable protein and nutrients to prevent aging. Select Asian mushrooms are slimming, high-protein foods. A few natural products have a romantic cachet. The calcium carbonate in pearl powder calms your nerves while it prevents and clears blemishes. Taken in capsules or used as a cream, it will make you feel as rare and valuable as a pearl.

Many of the remedies featured in *Healthy Beauty* will be new to you. In the Annotated Resource Guide, I introduce my favorite international mailorder and internet companies for natural health and beauty products. With them you will become familiar with a wide variety of products that include high fashion salons, healthfood stores, and Asian shops. I have drawn on knowledge from the world over to help you stay youthful and beautiful. I have offered alternatives such as homeopathic remedies where Asian herbs may not be easy to acquire. Convenience and price are always considerations. I describe quality natural products, which neither contain harmful ingredients nor are tested on animals.

At the other extreme, I include the latest medical findings on a variety of beauty-related issues. Each year I introduce medical doctors and nutritionists to the mysteries of New York City's Chinese and East Indian herbal markets during the annual conference "Botanical Medicine in Modern Clinical Practice" hosted by Columbia University's College of Physicians and Surgeons, The Rosenthal Center for Complementary and Alternative Medicine, University of Arizona's Department of Integrative Medicine, and New York Botanical Gardens. The conference features health professionals, including widely acclaimed author Dr. Andrew Weil, who share their enthusiasm for natural alternatives as well as their herb recipes. I have included exciting information inspired by Dr. Weil's research in my chapter on spot slimming. Obesity and diabetes are currently said to be epidemic in America. An eastern approach to health provides new avenues for beauty for both sexes.

The new American male is free to define himself and his looks according to who he wants to be—not what the job expects. Often there is no boss, just you at home wearing jockey shorts and a beard at your computer. Is it sexy? We think so. But sometimes, we want you to fix up and make us feel like lovers. In *Healthy Beauty*, you will get great advice from New York and Hollywood beauty and style professionals in a section called "Especially for Men" found in most chapters. It addresses questions ranging from the latest chic shaving cream and men's makeup to the best sources of herbal energy for work and play.

If you are not already in love, you probably will fall in love again. *Healthy Beauty* can help you to be ready. The pretty and handsome get admiring looks—and, the *New York Times* assures us, better pay. An "Economic Scene" column titled, "Like It or Not, Appearance Counts In the Workplace," reports on a study that found "better looking" American and Canadian lawyers got higher wages and faster promotions during the 1990s than their less attractive colleagues.

The world judges our appearance in its own terms. Turn on the television news, sports, or the market report: you will see a uniformly high standard of appearance. To mollify an exasperated stock trader, you need a vivacious

Maria Bartiromo, or a quietly sexy David Faber. To sit through the news of the latest flare-up in the Middle East, you need the smooth, reassuring voice of Leon Harris and the immaculate grooming of Paula Zahn or Daryn Kagan. Their relaxed, authoritative look is right on target. In the public eye, grooming counts.

The origin of healthy beauty runs deep. Its presence is arresting. Once in a London subway, I saw a woman who seemed to be a pre-Raphaelite portrait that had stepped out of its frame. Her face was a luminous pearl. Her reddish hair was cropped in bangs that approached the eyes. Her irregular features held me in awe. When I described this experience to handsome English actor Michael York, he remarked that, "Beauty is spiritual emanation rather than superficial appearance. We are all made of energy. Beauty is harmonious energy."

American Beauty

Driving through the lush New England countryside shortly after September 11, 2001, the leaves were bright yellow and red. Autumn hushed the swamp, where beavers lived under a river bank. A woolly Mongolian dog announced our arrival in a garden that overflowed with six foot high pink cleome and Himalayan impatiens. Pink, purple, and white phlox, yellow jewelweed, and violet echinacea grew near the billy goat's den. A comfrey patch spread near the nannies' house. The air had a Boursin fragrance. Our Vermont friends, a school principal and her tree surgeon husband, have provided us with goat milk for years. She, recently returned from China, wearing an elaborate Shanghai robe, officiated as Justice of the Peace at a commitment ceremony. The engaged couple had flown in two days earlier, leaving their acting jobs, Hollywood apartment, red convertible, and stuffed animals on their bed.

When the ceremony began, my loving partner of many years and I joined hands in a colorful, multiethnic circle that included friends, dogs, and goats. Someone recited an Apache wedding poem: "Now you will feel no rain, for each of you will be shelter to the other. Now you will feel no cold, for each of you will be warmth to the other. Now there is no loneliness for you." The couple exchanged vows and each promised, "When you are afraid, I will hold you in the dark. Though the world could end tomorrow, you and I will be together in whatever time we have. I will always love you." I gazed at a reflection of the wedding party in a nearby pool of water, whose clarity revealed our tribe of gay and straight, white, yellow, red, brown, and black Americans.

Once Narcissus fell in love with his mirror image in such a garden. The ancient Greeks loved beauty and considered it to be the highest truth. The simple and original ceremony we had witnessed held great promise for the future. Natural beauty is courageous because it accepts no boundaries for love. That year my darling mother, just turned 80, fell in love again. How wonderful that love is forever possible! The September 11th attack on our multicultural diversity—the world's trade center—has brought the nation closer. People have displayed the American flag from coast to coast. However, the time has come to acknowledge our true aesthetic: a rainbow of colors.

Healthy Beauty presents a practical approach to personal growth, a diary in which to mark your beauty and style changes. Healthy beauty is a statement of personal freedom that must be nurtured or else perish. Now more than ever, our appearance and well-being are threatened by stress, pollution, illness, and terrorism. This book celebrates a multicultural approach to beauty based on personal well-being. Those ready to accept the challenge can say, We *are* beautiful—free, united, and indestructible. Nothing veils our smile.

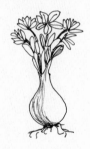

PART ONE

Healthy Narcissism

Who is the person in your mirror?

1

Your Mirror Image

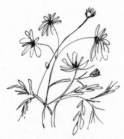

"Art, in a word, must not content itself simply with holding
the mirror up to nature, for it is a re-creation more than a
reflection, and not a repetition but rather a new song."
—OSCAR WILDE

Audrey Hepburn was nominated for an Academy Award for her portrayal of
Sister Luke in the 1959 Warner Brothers' movie *The Nun's Story*. The delicate 5'7" brunette, called "elf like" by reviewers, was loved for her elegance
and refinement. Sister Luke could not remain a nun for very long—she had a
bad habit of looking in a mirror. That was strictly forbidden because it inter-
rupted the necessary dialogue with God and began a dialogue with the self.
So-called vanity allowed for self-examination and change. Dressing without
looking in a mirror maintained order and conformity.

When was the last time you looked carefully at your naked body in a full-
length mirror? Try it. Are there aspects of you that you hardly recognize?
The ideal you dances in your imagination. It may be a younger or slimmer
or smoother face and body that you no longer can find. If you are the self-
critical type, your eye may magnify wrinkles or fasten on bulges. You become
certain your hairline is receding or jowl sagging. Is that a wart and was it there
before? No wonder you hesitate to spend time before the mirror. Its cool
objectivity threatens your inner, secret self.

Don't blame the mirror. You have the means to become an ever-evolving work of art. Looks change as habits improve. Mind, body, and spirit are parts of a complex energy system which is forever modifying itself to reflect good health or accommodate illness. The body is the surface of this profound whole. It shows the results of your diet, lifestyle, and emotional state. It is said that by 40 a person is responsible for his or her face. Life is demanding, yet beauty remains your birthright.

First, let's try to see ourselves from the outside, the way a stranger might. If the thought of getting naked in front of a stranger causes you some trepidation, try a homeopathic remedy. Easily available but not nearly as well-known in America as in Europe, homeopathics are often recommended to support emotional balance. The remedy is made from a refined, minute amount of a natural substance that, when placed under the tongue or added to drinking water, is absorbed quickly into the blood stream. Homeopathics do not require strong digestion. Any unnecessary portion of the remedy is easily eliminated from the body without side effects. However, never mix a homeopathic remedy with food and especially not with coffee. Even decaf coffee will cancel the remedy's effect, so wait at least one hour after drinking coffee before taking a remedy. Better yet, stay off the coffee altogether!

Healthy Beauty will target homeopathic remedies for specific beauty issues, such as a clear complexion or pleasant body odor. You can take one dose (5 pills) of gelsemium 30C to help you overcome the barrier of apprehension. This minute trace of yellow jasmine is recommended for conditions ranging from lethargy to stage fright or anxiety over a pending event, say a big date. It helps to settle the stomach and calm anxiety without acting as a sedative. An herbal alternative might be a warm cup of vervain or chamomile tea.

Your date here is with your mirror, preferably one full-length and multi-paneled, so you can see yourself from different angles.

See Yourself as Others Do

1. Stand undressed in front of a large mirror and place a hand over your eyes. Over your shoulder, peek at the curves, the trunk, the arms, hands, legs, and feet. Look at yourself from all angles.

What do you notice first? What areas need firming or reducing? Are there areas with cellulite or varicose veins? Enlarged veins may point to poor circulation. The regular use of homeopathic calcium (calcara fluoride 6x) can often improve circulation.

Is your back straight? Are your shoulders squared? Or do you find that one shoulder is higher than the other? Irregularities often point to fatigue or poor walking habits. We will address posture in Chapter 5, devoted to your walk.

Are there bulges at your waist or hips? Natural remedies and corrective diet and will help to firm your body and reduce impurities. Chapter 6, Spot Slimming, will zero in on problem areas.

Is your complexion clear and glowing, or dull and blemished? Where are acne, moles, birthmarks, or freckles located? The skin's condition indicates the health of digestion, elimination, and breathing. The chapters in Part Three will cover complexion and voice, describing ways to increase internal oxygen along with nutrients to brighten complexion.

2. Look at some of your recent photographs from all directions, including upside down, sideways, and backwards through the photograph. You will be able to see yourself in an entirely new way. Use a pencil to change the shape, size, style, or colors as you desire.

3. Cut out and post a photo of your ideal self. It might be someone in a fashion or health magazine that resembles your goal—an image of your desired look. You may like to draw or paint your ideal self. Make periodic visual notes of your progress.

Graphic artist Andy Warhol had his models pose for hundreds of photos in one-dollar picture booths so that he could see their many angles and moods. You might take a series once a month to watch your progress. Avoid a written diary. A diary is meant for a real or imagined audience. It can be used to persuade yourself of a change that isn't real. But pictures don't lie.

Hear Yourself as Others Do

1. Record your voice as you read from a book. Use a cassette recorder or even an answering machine. Is your voice clear, easy to understand, and relaxed, or is it strained and shrill? Listen to your voice recording from the next room. What picture does it conjure? What impression would your voice give to a stranger?

Try breathing deeper: stand straight and inhale gently into the lower abdomen without moving your chest. Let yourself relax and, to lengthen the breath, exhale as though it is through your legs and feet to the floor. Repeat this five times and record your voice again.

2. Stand close to a corner of your room. Cup your hands forward behind your ears and speak naturally. What you hear this way is close to what others hear. Is your voice high, trembling, breathy, groaning, or punctuated with staccato consonants? Or is it deep, rich, and melodious?

Energy and mood affect your voice. However, you will learn that your body or energy type (among the Chinese Five Elements: Fire, Earth, Metal, Water, and Wood) will also affect your voice. For example, a person considered to be an Earth type will have a voice that is sweet or singsong. Fatigue creates greater variations in pitch. Metal type people, whether or not they are singers, will occasionally require natural remedies to improve breathing and energy. You will learn ways to improve your breath capacity and vocal color in Chapter 16.

Perceive Your Fragrance as Others Do

Sniff an article of clothing that you have worn all day. Traditional Chinese doctors believe that distinctive body odors tell us something about our energy. When certain internal organs overwork from stress or poor habits, they give the body an unpleasant odor. Each odor is associated with one of the Five Elements. Here is a chart to summarize the relationship between odors, emotions and the Five Elements:

Odor	Emotion	Element
Bitter or burnt	Anxiety	Fire
Sweet or fetid	Worry	Earth
Metallic or pungent	Melancholy	Metal
Fishy or salty	Exhaustion, fear	Water
Sour or rotten	Anger	Wood

Note what your natural fragrance without deodorant reminds you of—something burnt, fragrant or sweet, coppery or metallic, fishy, or sour. It may be a combination of several aromas. Chapter 8 will inform you how to prevent unpleasant odors. It is always better to cleanse odors from the inside with diet and herbs rather than to apply a coverup. A neutral body fragrance indicates balance, whereas an odor signals inflammation or extreme emotions.

The rest of the book will help you to make improvements in the above areas and more. You will find detailed instructions for long-term prevention and treatment of beauty issues as well as Quick Fixes for immediate improvement. Above all, to succeed with your total makeover you need to accept your self-love, to work with it instead of denying it.

Healthy Narcissism

I have been intrigued by the Greek myth of Narcissus every since I first read the sexy parts of Ovid's *Metamorphoses* as a child. Later, studying to become a psychoanalyst in Paris, I began to quarrel with the traditional Freudian view that narcissism, or self-love, was a sign of arrested sexual development. In fact, Ovid's Narcissus loves not himself but an idealized version of himself, and his failure to embrace that vision causes him misery and death.

Recall that Narcissus was an especially beautiful young man with whom both men and women fell in love. Because he never reciprocated the feelings of others, the god Nemesis caused him to fall in love with a reflection of himself in a sylvan pool. He laments: "I am in love, and see my loved one, but that form which I see and love I cannot reach." However, Narcissus has a learning curve. Soon he declares: "Alas! I am myself the boy I see. I know it: my own reflection does not deceive me. I am on fire with love for my own self." This "self" is perfect—it will not age or become ill, it is always there just beyond reach. This is the imagined ideal self, which is based on your unique vision of personal beauty.

Radiant Health and Beauty

Healthy Narcissism is based on self-preservation and radiant health, not self-adoration. To be beautiful and vital, you must protect energy and immunity. The New Narcissus is informed, not only about style but about product safety. The current leading medicines for treating acne (Accutane) and hair loss (Rogaine) come with manufacturer's warnings against possible birth defects. Their use is forbidden during pregnancy. In a number of cases, other side effects from Accutane have included anxiety and suicidal depression. Even if the drugs themselves were not expensive, anxiety is too high a price to pay. Even if the drugs are discontinued, hair loss, acne, and anxiety symptoms return. Such medicines are not a final solution: they do not build healthy beauty or prevent illness and aging.

Unlike Narcissus, we need not pine away for our ideal self. We don't have to reach it completely, only to point ourselves in the right direction. The body and its good habits naturally improve when given the chance. Using natural remedies, we can move past self-love to self-improvement and self-expression in the most productive ways. We can all look and feel better for ourselves and others to admire. This I call Healthy Narcissism. Narcissus could neither love another person nor a non-ideal version of himself. He lacked generosity. The god Nemesis' ultimate revenge was that Narcissus was doomed to self-love without self-improvement.

Become a Trend-Bender

Do you accept a mirror image—a fashion trend—without blinking? If so, you need to start from square one to remake your look. One Saturday morning in Los Angeles, I enjoyed breakfast with Don Hill, the west coast business representative for Equity. It was in a Japanese garden restaurant where a waterfall emptied into a clear pool. Don, handsome, slim, and tall with polished American midwest manners, came dressed in casual black clothes and short brown hair. Privately, he is a health professional dedicated to eliminating physical discomforts and emotional blocks of his clients, including stunning models and actors. "It is amazing," he said, "they apologize for the first half hour about their weight and poor habits."

Don has his clients shut their eyes and inhale into the body that they were given, to accept themselves. Then they are free to relax and accept his treatment. His gorgeous clients are agitated because they have accepted not their *own* ideal self, but a standard of appearance established by the beauty and cosmetic industry, the print and film establishment, or society at large. "Trend-anxiety is major in L.A.," Don said. "The current ideal is the slim body of Brad Pitt and Tom Cruise. People apologize if they don't look like them. In the 1950s, everyone thought that Marilyn Monroe's full, opulent body was the most beautiful in the world. Today she might be considered *zaftig*. Most actresses' careers end at 40 unless they are willing to change." Don believes, "To change your appearance, you have to first accept yourself as you are then you can move on." Here is an exercise to get us started.

A Centering Exercise

Jin Shin Jyutsu is Japanese-inspired healing touch used to move blocked energy and balance emotions. We will use it to facilitate change. The following Jin Shin Jyutsu Central Line Hold can be done anytime you want to recharge energy.

Sit comfortably or lie flat on your back. Take relaxed breaths into your lower abdomen and close your eyes. Place four fingertips of your right hand at the center of the top of your head. An acupuncture point is located there that connects your front and back energy meridians.

Over a period of 10 or 15 minutes, move your left hand very slowly from the center of your forehead down the "central line" over the entire front of the trunk to touch the pubic bone. Feel the pulse from the right hand on top of your head and your left hand become balanced in warmth and pulse. You might hold to the count of 12 before moving your left hand downward to the next position. Without lifting them, glide the fingers of the left hand down the face to the nose, mouth, chin, neck, chest, and abdomen to the top of the pubic bone.

Points along the central line may be charged with emotions or feel empty. Wait there before moving on. When you reach the pubic bone with your left hand, move your right hand around so that the right fingers touch the coccyx (tailbone). One hand is placed in front and the other behind. Hold that position for as long as you want in order to recharge your "battery" in the pelvis.

Now, with an inner eye, see the ideal you—the way you want to look. Or enjoy the sensations of a younger, healthier, more beautiful you. If you are not yet ready, your vision will come in time. We have begun an ineluctable process.

The oldest and most widely used beauty remedy comes from the sea. Used throughout Asia, Latin America, and Europe and easily available in the United States, natural pearls heal body and mind. They are culled from the Persian Gulf to near Sri Lanka, Indonesia, the Gulf of Mexico, and even in the Mississippi River. You can find facial complexion soaps from Mexico made with pearl or mother of pearl sold at Rite Aid, CVS, or in the Latin American section of your local pharmacy.

In China, pearling has been known from before 1000 B.C. Powdered pearl, ingested with water as an anti-inflammatory herbal medicine or applied to the skin as a beauty treatment, was famously preferred by CiXi, the last Dowager Empress of China, during the Qing Dynasty. Her flawless complexion was renowned. The chief ingredient of powdered pearl, calcium carbonate ($CaCO_3$), can be absorbed orally or through the skin. Wing Hop Fung, the largest Chinese products store in Los Angeles, sells a beauty kit that contains pearl complexion cream and pearl powder. The powder combined with milk and honey makes a facial mask that speeds the skin's cell turnover. Dead cells are replaced with new skin. Pearl powder taken internally treats acne and reduces redness. It soothes dry eyes and eases insomnia, fever, and anxiety. The traditional uses of pearl demonstrate how health and beauty are intertwined. Improve your complexion with pearl and you will feel like smiling. Apply pearl creams, drink the powder added to water, and, if you can afford it, wear pearls in areas that benefit from its cooling influence (for example, around the neck or the left wrist or ankle). Traditional Chinese medicine considers the left side to be the side of the heart and our ocean of feelings. As we will see in the following chapter, the fine arts of beauty developed in European courts are no less worthy of attention.

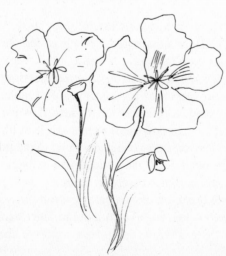

2

Lola's Way

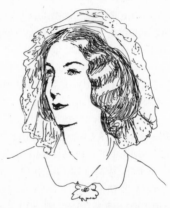

"A lady who dresses in such a manner as to attract attention to her dress is always badly dressed."
—LOLA MONTEZ

Is there a lace hat or tux hung in the back of your closet? Does a tennis racket
or a crumpled playbill lie hidden under a pair of old shoes? Before you can
improve your beauty, you may have to overcome a form of stage fright. Your
audience may be a crowded hall or simply your date for the evening. It is not
enough to be beautiful; you have to project beauty. Once I dreamed of a career
on the opera stage and starved myself to afford voice lessons. My closet
sequestered several elegant gowns. My ideal self had little to do with my student life at L'Ecole Normale de Musique in Paris. A talented and sophisticated
person longed to be born, but I had no idea how to begin.

My voice teachers promised a great career for me. I lived around the corner from the Louvre, yet I felt like a character from Puccini's *La Boheme*. My
hotel room contained a bed, a wall of full-length mirrors, a rented piano, and a

small sink in which I washed clothes, prepared dinner, and dyed my hair bright henna red. Away from home for the first time, I lacked security, comfort, and peace of mind. Each day, the large mirrors in my room forced me to confront the disparity between my actual and imagined selves. For the first time in my life, I felt alone and poor. If you don't live your dreams, they can destroy you.

Often I escaped to the Louvre, where I was inevitably drawn to Leonardo da Vinci's Mona Lisa. I found her comforting. Crowds of people from all parts of the globe stood hushed in worship. Her beauty secret is serenity. The Mona Lisa, who may be rich or poor, lover, wife, or mother, is in a state of harmony. I stared at her, while standing silent in the crowd. Despite my poverty I acknowledged an inner strength. Icons from classical art have a timeless quality that transcends appearance but appears beautiful. They evoke respect and lift your spirit because they tell a story.

Memorable beauty always evokes a story in the viewer. You have to set the scene with personal appearance and style. For example, the global appeal of Diana, the People's Princess, was inextricably associated with her good works. She would have made a great queen because she shared herself with her people. Her early vulnerability was overshadowed by fresh athletic appeal and royal elegance. You too create an impression each time you choose an outfit, walk, and speak. Is it one of nobility, efficiency, or some appealing aspect of your ethnic heritage? The quest for natural beauty is rewarding in itself. In this book, it is a path to freedom of imagination.

I never got around to storming the opera stage. Instead, I took up the banner of alternative medicine, which as it turned out called on my ability to perform. I found myself trading quips with Joan Rivers on radio, or doing traditional Asian diagnosis by examining the tongues of three soap opera stars on Donny and Marie's television show.

Overcome Stage Fright Naturally

To conquer my stage fright I learned a variety of techniques, including yogic breathing to quiet my nerves. To breathe calmly and deeply, stand with your feet shoulder width apart, inhale only into the lower abdomen, and exhale downward as though through your feet. Massage wrists and hands to help release tension in the chest. Step with one foot on to the top of the opposite foot to relax tension downward.

Attitude is very important for conquering nervousness. Luke Yankee, a leading theatrical director in Los Angeles, teaches at The American Academy of Dramatic Arts. He advises actors to prepare by "sending love and good will ahead to the audition." He says, "In a room of 300 actors at an open audition, the person that I, as a director, notice—the person whose energy jumps out and makes itself felt in a non-aggressive way—is centered and focused. That person owns the room. Everyone else fades." To achieve correct focus, Luke advises:

- Be gracious. Don't criticize others or make excuses for yourself.
- Be prepared: know your material.
- Be yourself.

You may never have an audition, but there are certainly times when you want to be noticed and admired! One way to be more beautiful is to smile. It worked for Mona Lisa. People can *feel* your message. A Japanese friend believes, "What makes a person beautiful is their interest in other people and enthusiasm for life." She adds, "Whoopi Goldberg's bright disposition and humor especially make her attractive, a pleasure to see and hear."

Lola's Way

Many historic figures have used advanced beauty skills to attain wealth and power. One inspiration for this book is Lola Montez, a nineteenth century *femme fatale* who became a countess and whose amazing book *The Arts of Beauty* I discovered at a used book stall on the banks of the Seine. As the world's first acknowledged beauty expert, her sound ideas and practical beauty recipes remain relevant to this day. She is the unacknowledged god-mother of today's natural beauty and cosmetic industry. Lola's recipes for baths, shampoos, creams, and lotions are made from herbs, foods, and mineral extracts. Because she urged her readers to make their beauty potions at home, we can still take advantage of them.

Lola rose to stardom in the Paris of Napoleon III, at a time when the City of Light was becoming the magnificent capital that we admire. The grand boulevards were under construction, soon to become lined by the familiar sidewalk cafés and the artistic life that went along with them. Lola was the first to perform modern interpretive dance. She captivated a crowd of famous, rich, and royal men. But above all, Lola became the first superstar— she was famous for being famous. People read about her in the two-penny newspapers and, in New York and London, flocked to her lectures on the fine art of being beautiful. From her lectures and best-selling book, we can enter an older world of elegance that still offers many practical hints on "the art of fascinating."

Sections labeled Lola's Way in subsequent chapters are inspired by her writing but have been brought up to date. They offer an alternative to our matter-of-fact world, where glamour has become commercial or tedious. Lola's Way presents an opportunity to fine-tune your personal aesthetics. Often herbal treatments are recommended along with activities meant to bring you closer to the beauty within. You can become an honorary count or countess if you wish to be.

Lola was born Eliza Gilbert in Limerick, Ireland, in 1818 to a young officer and his 13-year-old bride, who had escaped two months earlier from a convent school in order to become a dancer. Shortly afterward, the family moved to India, where the little girl admired court life among the maharajahs and maharanee. When Lola's father suddenly died, her mother returned Lola to a strict environment in Scotland. She arranged to marry her lovely teenager to a crusty old judge. Lola paid her back by eloping with Mom's boyfriend and returning to India to flaunt her new husband. The marriage did not last.

Back in London, Lola began Spanish dancing lessons. Making use of her pioneering sex scandals reported in *The London Times*, Lola headed for the Continent and fame. In 1844, Lola took up with the composer Franz Liszt, which he regretted. The same time, in Paris, two of her lovers killed each other in a duel. Lola's scandals were written about by Alexandre Dumas and Gustave Flaubert. A portrait of her done at this time shows a broad face with a clear, bright complexion, high cheekbones, a determined jaw, flashing dark eyes, and thick, wavy black hair. Her allure and style led to many romantic conquests.

Lola disdained artificial make-up. In *The Arts of Beauty*, she advises, "the great secret of acquiring a bright and beautiful skin lies in three simple things . . . temperance, exercise, and cleanliness. A young lady, were she as fair as a goddess, as charming as Venus herself, would soon destroy it all by too high living and late hours."

Lola, in keeping with the Eastern health traditions she had observed in India, advised against dietary extremes. She abhorred the customary European breakfast of strong coffee and hot buttered bread and a late dinner of "peppered soups, fish, roast, boiled, broiled, and fried meat, game, tarts, sweet-meats, ices, fruits, etc." She wrote that it would "derange the stomach (and) gradually overspread the fair skin with a wan or yellow hue." Eating richly and keeping late hours, she warned, would result in a shapeless, "flabby softness" we call cellulite. At the same time, "the once fair skin assumes a pallid rigidity or blotchy redness." We call that rosacea.

Basic beauty issues change little over the years. As the first beauty authority, Lola published secrets long cherished by the ladies of the courts of Europe. She had learned strange tricks. For example, women in the Spanish court improved the texture of their hands by sleeping with them elevated over their heads—they hung their arms from ropes embedded in the ceiling. Spanish ladies made their eyes shine by adding drops of Valencia orange juice. I have a better idea from an even more secretive court: apply soothing Chinese pearl drops as an eye wash. Several brands are easily available using the product resource section at the back of the book.

Lola's greatest conquest was King Ludwig I of Bavaria, who flipped for her when she burst into his bedchamber, cut her bodice strings, and danced naked for him. The elderly monarch built her a palace and Lola became the Countess of Lansfeld. The Catholic church was outraged. The queen wasn't too happy either. The king wrote love poems, while Lola ruled from the bed-chamber. The Revolution of 1848 dethroned both king and consort. However, we are not sad: in her brief, tumultuous life, Lola got what she wanted. The Harvard Theatre collection revealed a news clipping from an unnamed source: Lola Montez was "par eminence, the brilliant adventuress of this age and the last of that extraordinary class of talented, emancipated women which has been a puzzle and a grief to the disbelievers in woman's capacity for bold thought and free action."

Lola Montez grasped the eternal secrets of beauty and style. "The object of dress should be to show off an elegant woman," she wrote, "and not an elegantly dressed woman." What we add to our natural gifts must express our ideal self.

Especially for Men

Lola Montez wrote "Hints To Gentlemen on the Art of Fascinating" as part of *The Arts of Beauty*. Her rules of conduct for a lover are often ironic. The first was: "Make yourself as big a fool as possible, in order to ensure the most speedy and triumphant success." Lola berates men who flirt or ogle people in public. However, I think that skillful flirting is essential in creating appeal in either sex.

In New York, I've noticed that men often flirt by clearing their throat or opening their eyes wider when they see a pretty woman. I suppose it's a safety measure—a subtle move in case the woman is not interested. A person may vaguely complain about something inconsequential such as the weather to see if a potential lover responds. Although it can be a low-impact conversation opener, it could sadly end up as a mutual complaint session.

If you are charming and polite, your opener need not be believable. A mature, celebrated Italian professor once introduced himself to me, a student, at a university conference in Urbino. When he heard my name he said, "A col-league told me that a particularly beautiful Hungarian woman would be here tonight. He is a friend of hers and he asked me to protect her. That must be you," he said as he smiled. I smiled back and he protected me for some time.

Flirting Basics

- Notice and mention the person's positive or beautiful features.
- Pay a polite compliment suited to the situation.
- It is okay to exaggerate praise if it's done with good intentions.
- Have fun but don't be a pest. Wait for eye contact or an answer before continuing.

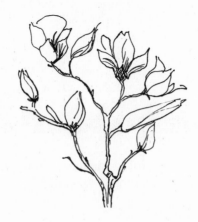

3

Stress Fighters

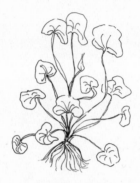

"Youth and age are partly a matter of habit and training."
—*PERSONAL RENEWAL*

Stress is aging and uglifying. Worse, it's physically unavoidable. Back when we lived in caves, gathered roots and berries, and first discovered green tea (about 3500 B.C.), when faced with a wild boar or saber-toothed tiger, our body reacted immediately. Heart rate increased to supply oxygen for the heart, lungs, and muscles. Blood pressure increased as circulation was redirected. Blood coagulability increased to protect against bleeding to death from possible wounds. Protection against shock left the skin clammy, shivering, and goose-fleshed to conserve body heat. We began to sweat. Breathing accelerated. Eyes opened wide, with pupils dilated. The body tensed as adrenalin, noradrenalin, and hormonal support readied us to spring into action.

At that point we had two choices—run away screaming or use a natural remedy. Our stressors have changed over time, but our body remains genetically programmed to react as though we never left the cave. In the middle of a heart-pounding panic attack, you may fear imminent death. Your body is protecting you from an unseen stressor. By defining stress, it becomes manageable. Like naming a demon, you can take a deep breath and say to yourself,

"It's just the old fight-or-flight syndrome." Then use what works for you—meditation, prayer, or visualizing a calmer situation—so that you can move forward. My way of dealing with stress is to plan for it.

What Herbal Stress Fighters Can Do

Herbs provide a powerful way to reduce stress and protect appearance. You need not buy exotic ingredients to take advantage of ancient herbal wisdom. Once you accept that herbs, foods, and teas can enhance vitality, you can use the herbal tradition you know. Well-chosen Asian herbs, Western health-food store products, or East Indian, Latin American, or African herbs work wonders regardless of your national origin. Herbs are rejuvenating. Because they are absorbed like foods, herbs work as catalysts to stimulate necessary physical reactions such as digestion, respiration, and elimination of toxins.

Basic Definitions

Several categories of herbs for internal use are important for you to know. They are herbal cleansers, tonics, and adaptogens. The following foods and herbs for daily use can create a baseline for health and balance required for beauty. They will improve weight-loss and anti-addiction programs, improve resistance to colds and flu, and enhance vitality. Specific remedies covered in Chapter 17, Beauty Survival Skills, will help protect against injury and terrorism.

Herbal Cleansers: Protection from Bad Habits and Pollution

A household cleanser or bleach kills germs and eliminates stains. An herbal cleanser for internal use such as a tea, liquid tincture, or pill eliminates acids, unabsorbed foods, or other impurities. Often cleansing is accomplished by naturally increasing urination, bowel movements, or sweating. You can use herbal cleansers to eliminate blemishes and reduce water retention. Most frequently they are bitter-tasting plants and green or yellow vegetables such as chicory, endive, and squash.

Dandelion or tarragon increase bile flow. Bile is laxative, extremely bitter, green-colored, and alkaline. It speeds digestion and cleanses impurities from the blood. After using a stimulant cleanser, the body feels lighter and cleaner and complexion is smoother. Other herbal cleansers include parsley and cilantro, which are diuretic (increase urination), and rhubarb, which is laxative.

After eating cleansing foods, we feel cool and refreshed because they remove excess acid. I have seen plenty of people who have dry red eyes, acne, flaky and itchy rough skin, thinning hair, dry cough, stomach ulcers, constipation, bad breath, nervousness, or other signs of inflammation, but who continue to gorge themselves with hot spices, salt, alcohol, sugar, and greasy foods, as well as to smoke cigarettes. For picante eaters, using cooling herbs and spices such as cumin, coriander, and fennel seeds, mint, dill, cilantro, alfalfa, cucumber, zucchini, or spinach might seem a revolutionary dietary and lifestyle change. Without cooling, cleansing foods, their beauty will suffer. They will be troubled by stress, nervousness, and insomnia, which are increased by acid.

Traditional Chinese medicine's energetic point of view has become an international language shared by European and American herbalists as well as the Chinese. Laboratoire 5 Saisons located in Aix-en-Provence, France, makes Elixir Energetic #2 (Depurgatif Fois), a concentrated liquid-extract liver cleanser that contains sirop d'erable (maple) as a source of calcium, magnesium, phosphorus, and manganese as well as romarin (rosemary), verbenone (vervain), pissenlit (dandelion), gattilier (*Agnus castus*), cimicifuga (black cohosh), chelidoine (celandine), and alchemille (lady's mantle). The line of ten energetic elixirs is formulated by noted French author and educator Dr. Yves Requena, who though trained as a Western endocrinologist practices traditional Chinese medicine.

Herbal Tonics Replenish What Age and Illness Have Depleted

A tonic is a food that helps the body to work better. Often we use a tonic to increase energy and endurance (for example, Chinese ginseng). Herbs with stimulating properties such as sage or nettle also stimulate energy and increase immunity to illness or fatigue. Asian tonics are sometimes semi-sweet fruits or fungi (the mushroom family), also roots, twigs, bark, shells, or animal products.

Herbal tonics stimulate and nourish the body differently than vitamins. An herbal blood-enhancing tonic such as shu di huang (*Rehmannia glutinosa*) does not contain iron but improves the health of the liver and kidney, which are vital to blood production. Bing cherry concentrate, often used to reduce gout pains, supplies minerals that condition the liver. An herbal tonic does more than supplement nutrition, it stimulates organ functions.

Use a stimulating herbal energy tonic if you look and feel rundown, your complexion is pale and dull, your movements are slow and clumsy, and you feel weak and achy. A blood-enhancing tonic such as dong quai (*Angelica sinensis*), also known as tang kuei, is sometimes recommended after a menstrual period if you feel chilled and washed out. Otherwise, a blood tonic such as bing cherries is good anytime because it is nutritious and cleansing. I like adding two or more tablespoons of Dr. Bernard Jensen's Bing Cherry Concentrate to water first thing in the morning or as a mid-afternoon energy lift. Add sparkling water and a dash of lemon for tart flavor.

Nerve tonics (sometimes called nervines) are rejuvenating for people who think constantly, who break out in nervous rashes or suffer from nerve pains (neuralgia and sciatica), who lie awake at night unable to remember things, or who age mentally from stress. Among this respected category of tonics is an Asian star, gotu kola. Dr. Vasant Lad in *The Yoga of Herbs*, a book reread to shreds in my library, writes that gotu kola (*Hydrocotyle asiatica*) is recommended for "senility, premature aging, hair loss, chronic and obstinate skin conditions (such as eczema, psoriasis and leprosy!), and that it may be the most important rejuvenative herb in Ayurvedic (East Indian) medicine."

A lovely man originally from Puna, India, Dr. Lad once opened an herb class I attended by singing from the *Vedas* about *prana* (the flow of life) in Sanskrit. I was totally charmed. About gotu kola he writes, "It increases intelligence, longevity, memory; it decreases senility and aging. It fortifies the immune system, both cleansing and feeding it, and strengthens the adrenals." Founder and director of the Ayurvedic Institute in Albuquerque, Vasant Lad has penetrating, warm eyes and an easy, friendly manner. He writes well-researched, comprehensive, and charming books. When it comes to advice on nerve tonics, which impact on mind and spirit, it pays to consider the source.

Adaptogens Reduce Wear and Tear

Adaptogens are a special category of tonics used to prevent fatigue and illness resulting from stress and weakened immunity. In later chapters, you will learn how to choose the right ginseng and mushroom for weight loss as well as for performance strength and endurance.

Japanese mushrooms such as shiitake, reishi, and enoki are famous sources of polysaccharides—very large, long-chain sugar molecules that are structural components of many cells. Polysaccharides are active compounds in a number of medicinal plants and foods that are nontoxic but have powerful enhancing effects on immunity. They increase "natural killer cells," which are the main destroyers of malignant cells, as well as increased resistance to invasion of bacteria and viruses. Mushrooms such as shiitake, oyster mushrooms, enoki, and maitake are a delicious way to protect vitality and reduce stress.

Merely knowing how healthy mushrooms are gives us reason for pause. They have survived dinosaurs, world wars, and human environmental stupidity. According to Paul Stamets in *Mycomedicinals: An Informational Booklet on Medicinal Mushrooms,* "The 5300-year-old Ice Man who was discovered in the fall of 1991 on the border of Austria and Italy packed three polypore species with him, implying that he considered them essential to his trek over the Alps." Polypores are conk-shaped mushrooms that grow attached to trees and have pores underneath instead of gills. This cave woman also uses ling zhi (reishi) and shiitake.

Adding generous amounts of cooked medicinal mushrooms to diet protects us from health worries. That alone is rejuvenating! Asian mushrooms are often used as combination liquid extracts to combat environmental poisons and infection. Numerous Asian studies reported by distinguished authors and educators such as Dr. Andrew Weil and Paul Stamets suggest that the benefits of medicinal mushrooms reach far beyond their taste or any possible placebo effect.

Medicinal Mushrooms and Beauty

The cleansing, anti-inflammatory actions of Asian mushrooms also prevent blemishes, rosacea, hair loss, wrinkles, excess weight, cholesterol-related poor circulation, grouchiness, and stress insomnia. That sounds like aging. Medicinal mushroom extracts are especially useful for students, athletes, dancers and performers, executives, and media personalities, and for jet travel. When you need endurance and peak energy, you especially need their strong protection. Because they have many uses, I will discuss them throughout this book. The following chapter describes mushrooms suited for every season and weather condition.

Stress always shows on the face. The more caffeine you consume, the more tired and wrinkled you look. With less coffee and chocolate, the face is fuller and the complexion brighter. Your hair does not fill the comb. A medicinal mushroom tea can ease craving for sweets. Mushrooms protect and nourish every fiber of your being.

I cook medicinal mushrooms in a crockpot set at a low setting for four to eight hours and drink the juice, which resembles a foamy, bitter-tasting beer. You can sweeten it by adding dried figs while cooking. I often add some of the appropriate ginseng to cook with medicinal mushrooms because their energies are complementary. For example, I cook ling zhi (reishi), an anti-inflammatory mushroom useful for arthritis, along with raw tienchi ginseng, a cooling ginseng that increases circulation and reduces pain.

Using a commercial mushroom liquid extract is convenient for work and travel. You can take 40–60 drops daily in water, wine, or juice. Persons dealing with immune-threatening disease, high stress, frequent jet travel, or who are at risk of environmental poisons should use a combination of mushrooms such as Stamets 7 Mushroom Blend, formulated by Paul Stamets. He, the author of several beautifully illustrated and carefully researched books, teaches classes in growing gourmet and medicinal mushrooms at his laboratory Fungi Perfecti in Washington State (see www.fungi.com). Long Hay Flat makes a highly concentrated mushroom extract called Reishi+ for energy, endurance, and immune enhancement. The dose is 3–5 drops twice daily. Read about their products in the Quick Fix section of this chapter.

Some people prefer capsules. Intelligent Choice, located in Los Angeles, supplies Japanese health foods to hospitals. Their website www.absolutely healthy.com sells fine Japanese consumer health products. For stress management, Pristine, their line of concentrated food capsules, includes Ashitaba root used to treat diabetes and stress acne, and Suppon Japanese turtle shell (cooling and moistening), which increases stamina, improves sleep, and clears acne blemishes. LEM is a concentrated extract of shiitake, one of the world's most highly praised and researched mushrooms, used to boost immunity to illness and chronic fatigue, balance blood sugar, and reduce cholesterol.

Skip Ishii is the dynamic CEO for Intelligent Choice as well as several Los Angeles health-food companies. Originally a television producer in Japan and author of a book (in Japanese) on how to thrive in the United States, he and his family are doing the L.A. thing. Skip educates American consumers about the benefits of traditional Japanese foods. Japan has the largest population in the world of those aged 100 years and older.

Cordyceps sinensis

Cordyceps, one of the most popular medicinal fungi from Asia, has potent adaptogenic qualities and is available in Chinese herb shops and on the internet. It maintains daily wellness and is suited to any sort of travel. I will discuss remedies for anxiety in Chapter 17.

Cordyceps (dong chong xia cao) looks like a small dried worm. The empty pod left by a caterpillar, cordyceps takes the shape of its former tenant, sort of like the shell that remains after a snail leaves. Chinese herbalists value it highly as an anti-tumor and immuno-stimulant herb. Laboratory tests reported by Paul Stamets confirm many other important uses. For example, the species has cholesterol-reducing and general cardiotonic properties. Hot-water extracts contain compounds that relax the bronchial passages, easing breathing. Cordyceps also dilates the aorta by 40% when we are under stress. The increased blood flow benefits muscles pushed to the max and increases endurance. A clinical study done in 1985 with sexually dysfunctional men found that 64% improved in performance from ingesting 1 gram per day. Another clinical study in 1995 reported that 36 patients with advanced breast and lung cancer had "restored cellular immunological function" from cordyceps. A study done in 1994 found that cordyceps helped prevent kidney disease. Cordyceps has liver-fortifying actions and has been effective for improving hepatic function for Hepatitis B. The findings implicate that cordyceps has great value as a general nerve tonic.

Cordyceps, a super stress fighter, improves your looks, mood, and performance. Fatigue and dehydration age the skin, and increase falling hair, brittle nails, dark circles around the eyes, an ashen pallor, and a lackluster appearance. Asian herbal tonics such as cordyceps do more than cover up complexion problems: they prevent them.

Chinese chefs add a handful of cordyceps to improve the flavor of chicken or duck soup. You might add medicinal mushrooms such as cordyceps, ling zhi, and shiitake to leftover chicken bones along with a piece of dong quai and no salt. Simmer this at low heat for several hours in order to make a nourishing, tangy soup stock. For convenience, I recommend taking 20–30 drops of cordyceps extract on a regular daily basis to avoid collapse from jet travel, overwork, and the inevitable sabertooth tiger.

Anti-Stress Bodywork

Sitting on board an aircraft or simmering from stress at an office desk, our movements are limited. There are a few finger-pressure points located on the arms and hands that you can use to redirect energy flow and help relieve anxiety.

Anxiety makes the heart pound and breath short, causing panting. To relax the upper body and deepen breath, sit comfortably in a chair placing your hands at your navel. Inhale slowly only into the lower abdomen. Exhale from the lower abdomen through your legs to the floor.

Cross your arms on your chest and place your middle finger into the crook of the L at the opposite elbow. Found where the arm makes a right angle, it feels like a crevice where the elbow joint moves. If you can't find it, put the palm of one hand on the top and front of your opposite shoulder. Slide it down from shoulder to elbow. The point is under your palm where the elbow bends.

Push firmly with each middle finger into the crevice at the L. That releases stress stuck in the sinus area, head, neck, and upper arm. It is an acupuncture point used to bring inflammation from the head downward toward the fingers. Inhale, and as you exhale, press deeper at each elbow.

Now, release the arm, turn each palm upward and find the line of each inner wrist. There are located points that help reduce stress from the heart and pericardium. With the thumb press the inner wrist of the opposite hand until you can breathe deeper. Often one area of the inner wrist will appear red or inflamed. The area of the inner wrist nearest to the little finger corresponds to the heart. Applying pressure there helps to moderate heart action and reduce

panic. I press that point on both wrists for temporary relief from chest discomfort and to help improve insomnia.

Finally, hold the index finger of the left hand with the right four fingers.
Extend the right thumb and press hard with the thumb into the area between
the angle of the thumb and index finger of the left hand. Hold the position for
the count of 50 and switch sides. The left hand holds the right index finger
as the left thumb pushes (hoku) an acupuncture point that eases stress and
reduces pain.

Health and Beauty Maintenance

You need to take extra precautions with the change of seasons or when traveling to a different climate. All stress ages complexion and reduces vitality.
Here is an easy way to observe what teas and foods you will need to use.

Your Tongue Mirrors Vitality and Digestion

Traditional Asian doctors always observe the tongue as an indication of vitality. Its shape and color indicate the presence or absence of inflammation,
weakness, as well as circulation throughout the body. Observe your tongue
daily when you awaken and later in the day to note changes in energy and
metabolism. Observe it when you are confused about your diet choices or the
effects of pollution and weather conditions. Observing your tongue will begin
an ongoing relationship with your evolving beauty persona.

To observe your tongue in a mirror, use bright, indirect lighting. Relax.
Let your tongue hang like a dog panting in order to maintain its proper shape.
Notice its color, shape, and any markings such as a coating, spots, cracks and
bulges. The body of the tongue is a guide to long-term health and beauty
issues. The coating indicates temporary reactions to foods being digested.

Travel, especially to a different climate, compromises vitality and looks.
You might fly from New York to the tropics or from the countryside to a polluted city. Stagnant air in flight and smoke-filled rooms dull complexion, fraz-
zle hair, and scorch nerves. If your tongue trembles when you observe it, a
sign of chronic nervous tension or liver stress, your reactions to climate,
travel, and pollution will be stronger than for other people. Here are other
things to notice while looking at your tongue.

A Coated Tongue

A thick coating indicates slow or difficult digestion and mucus congestion,
which can affect digestion, breathing, joint comfort, and mental clarity. To
reduce mucus, eat more cleansing foods like barley soup and digestive herbs

such as a tea made with ginger and mint. Avoid overly sweet, sticky, heavy, and oily or fried foods and beer. A thick white, yellow, gray, or green tongue coating will often indicate nausea and food retention. "Spring cleansing" with foods and herbs is required no matter what the season. Don't eat heavily during long flights and take extra digestive herbs. I often take along apples and a thermos of green tea.

A Puffy Tongue

During travel, we tend to retain excess fluids. If your tongue is puffy and water-logged, a sign of slow metabolism and low energy, cleansing herbs normally used for humid languid weather such as dandelion will reduce water retention. A humid climate requires laxative and diuretic (cleansing) herbs that cleanse the liver. They perk up energy and enthusiasm, while reducing ingestion, bloating, puffy skin tone, and blemished complexion. Homeopathic natrum sulphate 6x (sodium sulphate) is recommended to ease digestion and breathing problems made worse by humid weather and rich foods.

In the tropics (hot, humid weather), avoid heavy or oily facial creams and moisturizers that clog pores.

A Pale Tongue

A pale tongue can correspond with weakness, chills, or poor endurance. It may be more frequent during wet, cold weather, but can also persist from overwork or a diet of too many cold raw foods and iced drinks. If tongue and gums are very pale, often a sign of anemia, you may require additional nutritional support and stimulant herbs such as sage tea or Chinese ginseng normally recommended during convalescence or in a harsh, cold climate. An energy tonic can boost energy and lift spirits.

In a cold climate, use a facial moisturizer or night cream, depending on your skin type. The moisturizer will help your body to hold in moisture and warmth.

A Red Tongue

A reddish, dry tongue can correspond with inflammation resulting from smoking, drinking, or eating spicy foods. It can indicate chronic conditions such as hypertension, diabetes, or menopausal symptoms. If your tongue is dry, red, and cracked, a sign of internal dehydration or inflammation, add more cooling green vegetables and avoid hot spices in order to reduce irritations, rashes, and bloodshot eyes. Homeopathic iron in the form of ferrum phosphate 6x is always useful in cases of inflammation and blood deficiency.

To help prevent dry skin, wrinkles, and rosacea (broken facial capillaries), spray your face with pure rose water and avoid all facial products that contain alcohol. In the desert, use a rejuvenating moisturizer such as Georgette Klinger's Skin Booster with Vitamin C or Jason Natural Cosmetics' line of Super C skin products. Creams and lotions that contain Ester C are anti-inflammatory and recommended to slow signs of aging.

Without Sleep, Beauty Is Lost

There are many causes for insomnia, including anxiety, hunger, and inflammatory conditions from blood and moisture deficiency. We will look at these and related issues throughout the book. However, one quick, effective remedy is homeopathic Calms Forte. It is made from a combination of minerals such as iron, calcium, potassium, and magnesium as well as relaxing herbs such as hops, that can reduce the underlying causes of nervous insomnia and restlessness. The dosage is 1–2 tablets as needed during the day or evening.

A Quick Fix Anti-Stress and Energy Tonic

Long Hay Flat brand Chinese herb supplements available from East Earth Trade Winds in Redding, California (www.eastearthtrade.com) makes a number of highly concentrated liquid extracts that are easy to carry in your purse or pocket. Among single herbs, Schizandra berry extract has been shown to strengthen and quicken reflexes and improve visual acuity. It curbs excess sweating and energy loss to fortify beauty and vitality over time.

My favorite Long Hay Flat combination extracts are Energy, Gentle Rejuvenator, Soothing Balance, and Supernourishing Extract. Here is a quick reference chart for their use and recommended dosage:

Product	Tonic Actions	Dose as Needed
Energy	Mental clarity	3–5 drops
	Physical energy	6–12 drops
Gentle Rejuvenator	Moistening, anti-aging	10–20 drops
Soothing Balance	Digestion, anti-depression	10 drops
Supernourishing Extract	Fatigue, sweet tooth	10 drops

Especially for Men

Damiana (*Turnera diffusa*) provides a generally stimulating and enhancing influence on the male reproductive system. According to Simon Mills, director of the Centre for Complementary Health Studies at Exeter University and author of the excellent, carefully researched, and gracefully written book, *Out of the Earth,* damiana's alkaloids are thought to have a testosteronal effect (similar to sarsaparilla) and contain constituents similar to those of caffeine. Other glycosides in the herb provide a relaxing influence. It is a stimulant that does not increase stress.

The shrub grows in Texas, Mexico, and Central American and is used by Native American women to increase sex drive after menopause. They may be attracted to the herb's adrenal stimulant qualities. It also makes a nice bitter aromatic tea.

The herb has been used by both sexes as an aphrodisiac and herbal euphoric. It improves stamina and mood as a tonic for the central nervous system. Simon Mills has written, "Damiana may be recommended in any debilitated condition of the central nervous system (from depression to neuralgias and problems such as herpes—it has a particular use in containing genital herpes). Although male-oriented it is not contra-indicated for women with debilitated conditions: its main contra-indications are in the very excitable and those with irritable bowel syndrome. Otherwise, it often fills a desirable place in a prescription for those simply too *sad*."

The dosage Mills recommends is 1–4 grams of the dried herb or the equivalent taken for a total of three times daily either in an infusion (tea) or a tincture made with 60% alcohol. That translates into approximately 30–90 drops of alcohol-based extract or 3–4 capsules (1520 mg) three times daily.

Lola's Way

Lola Montez believed that we preserve beauty best by making products such as lotions, creams, and shampoos at home. One way to defeat stress is a fine old European custom—making medicinal wines and liquors at home. Here is a tasty liquor made from a famous Chinese herbal blood-enhancing tonic. It requires no special equipment to make. (Avoid alcohol during pregnancy.) Liquor is by nature warming. If your complexion is ruddy, avoid alcohol and make the ingredients into a tea or add no more than 10 drops of the extract to a cooling beverage such as aloe vera juice or apple juice.

Skin Glow Spritzer

This is a sweet spicy liquor you can add 20 or 30 drops at a time to sparkling water or fruit juice. It perks up a tired complexion. The fruit ingredients nourish blood. Dong quai is a famous spicy sweet-tasting Chinese tonic suggested for balance and harmony.

Ingredients:
1 liter of vodka

One cup of a dried fruit such as figs, sweet cherries, peaches, or prunes
One dong quai root (*Angelica Sinensis*)

If you plan to consume the finished liquor within one week after decanting, you might use vermouth, which contains 18% alcohol, or brandy, which
contains 40% alcohol. A higher alcohol content assures freshness for a longer
time.

Thoroughly wash the dried fruit by placing it in a pot of water, covering
it, and bringing it to a boil. Steep it for a few minutes and pour off the water.
Rinse with clean water. Pat the fruit dry and slice it if necessary. In the same
way, wash one piece of dong quai.

Place the washed fruit and dong quai root into a decanter and fill it with
liquor, leaving 1 inch at the top of the bottle so that the fruit can expand. Leave
this in a cool, dry place for one to two weeks. Steeping it longer may make it
taste bitter. Enjoy this anytime you do not have a fever. It is warming, satisfying, and enlivening. Although dong quai is often recommended for fatigue
and a dull, pale complexion after menstruation, men can enjoy it too.

Both men and women are called on to work, travel, and compete with the
best in their profession. The following chapter will help your beauty bloom
in any climate.

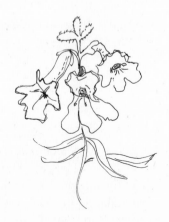

4

Your Seasons of Beauty

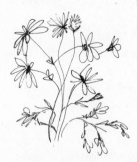

"The frequent and sudden changes in this country from
heat to cold, by abruptly exciting or repressing the
secretions of the skin, roughen its texture, injure its hue,
and often deform it with unseemly eruptions."
—LOLA MONTEZ

Beauty flourishes with a fresh face for each season. A few highly successful restaurants know this. Among New York's class acts, The Four Seasons has been famous since it opened in 1959. Managers Alex von Bidder and Julian Niccoli confer with their chefs for a menu that varies with each season. In spring, you will find soft-shell crabs, snow peas, fiddlehead ferns, beets, and sugar snap beans; in fall and winter, game with truffles and root vegetables. We ought to vary our diet in order to assure the best beauty results. Energy needs are seasonal and should be supplied by variety, the spice of cuisine.

The climate of your home town and vacation or business destination will also affect your energy, mood, and complexion. When you need to look your best, you don't want to fight the climate. Lola Montez recommended wearing a large bonnet to protect complexion from atmospheric assaults. In this chapter, I recommend teas and foods to fit your local climate or travel destination so that you can look and feel your best anywhere.

Your Personal Forecast

It is essential to acknowledge your individual needs over other considerations. You can determine a visual baseline for beauty and vitality by observing your tongue daily as you did in Chapter 3. Barring illness, here is a chart that will keep your energy on track and prevent most breakouts, allergies, and other problems affected by weather and travel.

Climate Stress, Pollution, and Beauty

Here is a handy guide just to remind you of the right foods and remedies for each season and climate. You will read more about them throughout the rest of the book.

Use Herbal Cleansers and Toners
When: in Spring and Summer (in North America)
If: Humid, warm weather or bad habits slow internal cleansing
Your tongue looks red, purple, swollen, coated, or spotted
Use:
- Bitter cleansing herbs: dandelion, skullcap, prunella, chicory, and endive in salads; gentian extract in water before meals
- Yin/Yang Sisters Instant Beverages as needed, including: Clean Habits, Get Svelte!, and Happy Garden Tea
- Zhu ling or ling zhi mushrooms, or Stamets 7 Mushroom Blend combination mushroom extract

Use Herbal Tonics and Adaptogens
When: in Fall and Winter (in North America)
If: Cold weather, jetlag, overwork, and upset drain vitality
Your tongue looks pale, scalloped, or quivering
Use:
- Semi-sweet and warm herbs: ginger, astragalus, dong quai, Chinese ginseng; calming herbs: Siberian ginseng tea
- Yin/Yang Instant Beverages as needed, including: Adapto-Gin, Breathe Free, Gorgeous You, Flu Away, or Romantic High
- Shiitake, cordyceps, or Stamets 7 Mushroom Blend

The Five Climates of Beauty

Ancient Chinese doctor-philosophers believed that we are made of the same stuff as all things on earth and in heaven. Humans—made metaphorically of fire, earth, metal, water, and wood—are part of Nature and subject to her influence. Wind, cold, heat, dryness, and humidity affect the quality of skin and hair as well as energy level.

Each season has beauty challenges and opportunities. Hot and dry weather or radiator heat withers hair and skin. Humidity makes energy droop and digestion suffer so that we are likely to gain pounds and retain water. Cold weather drains our color and warmth. However, you can compensate for this by using the right foods and herbs.

The following foods and teas made with cooking spices and garden herbs harmonize energy and prevent beauty problems. Enjoy them whenever and wherever you may be in a similar climate. You will make progress faster when daily discomforts are eased. The recommendations are safe for everyone. With care, you can eat them as needed for chronic beauty issues associated with a particular climate. I refer to seasons in North America with the understanding that your climate may vary. For that reason, I include weather conditions.

Spring: Humidity, Pollution, High Winds, or Allergy Season
Influence: Liver, gallbladder, muscles, nerves, and vision
Issues: Detoxification—blemishes, aches, and allergies

Spring in North America is a season of humidity, winds, and liverish problems such as allergies and headaches. Humidity can make your life miserable no matter where you are. Inflammatory conditions, water retention, mucus congestion, abdominal bloating, and sinus allergies become worse. Skin rashes and aches tend to be problematic. Mucus is the body's natural reaction to irritants. Ask anyone about their springtime allergies and they will complain about thick, yellow, green, or odorous discharges from eyes, nose, and ears. Pollen, dust, and fur allergies often increase in spring. Allergies harm appearance. Besides, your friends don't want to be sneezed on! Cleansing and balancing spring tonics ease stress.

Constipation allows acids to irritate and acne to increase. Many of the following cleansing spring foods and herbs are rich in minerals such as potassium, calcium, and silicea, which support healthy skin, hair, and fingernails.

Cleansing Teas and Beverages

Cumin, Coriander, and Fennel Seed Tea Stop Heartburn

These three kitchen spices remove acidity and inflammation from the digestive tract. Many springtime allergies and skin blemishes can be prevented with this cleansing tea. It works great for PMS water bloating, anxiety, and pains. Cumin is useful to prevent stomach ulcers, and therefore bad breath. Coriander is diuretic for thick, dark, or burning urination. It reduces water retention in the middle and legs. Fennel seeds, often offered as a digestive snack in East Indian restaurants, are digestive and help reduce bloating.

For sweeter breath and fewer complexion blemishes, make an anti-acid tea by adding ¼ teaspoon of each powdered spice to 1 cup of hot water. Drink it once or twice daily after a meal. The effect will be soothing, laxative, and diuretic. You may notice that acid burns or looks orange as it comes out in wastes. It is better to get rid of excess acid. If you suffer from chronic acid reflux, bad breath, constipation, or skin rashes, use this tea daily for at least one week before proceeding with other teas.

I also recommend nettle and yellow dock teas for beauty. Nettle, usually considered an adrenal tonic and blood-cleansing herb, improves hair condition and reduces allergies. Yellow dock is an excellent lymph cleanser, traditionally recommended for complexion because it improves the iron content of blood as well as enhances circulation. Both herbs are rich in minerals and easy to find in pharmacies and healthfood stores everywhere.

Cleansing Fruits and Vegetables

Spring and summer are great times to lose weight because we can enjoy many tasty raw fruits and vegetables. Increase healthy fun foods. Watermelon makes a delicious breakfast or snack that is high in potassium. It reduces blemishes, inches, dark circles around the eyes, and fatigue. Raw apples and celery make a nice spring breakfast (or pre-breakfast) because they clear mucus congestion while they tend to reduce cellulite and cholesterol. They are cleansing and laxative. I enjoy them with a pot of hot green tea. Apples' pectin is slimming because it has the ability to absorb excess water in the intestines. Apple fiber is non-irritating if you peel apples. The iron in apples is not high but it helps the body to absorb the iron in other foods. Apples contain a generous amount of vitamin C and calcium, and 50% more vitamin A than oranges. For that reason apples can protect eye beauty and vision.

Celery is high in roughage and low in calories. Its water content makes it especially good to eat with heavy starches. It is alkaline, which helps to protect the body from acid irritations. The greener stalks of celery are a good source of vitamins A, B1, and G. It is rich in chlorine, natural sodium, potassium, and magnesium. These minerals improve joint comfort and enhance a graceful walk.

Other helpful vegetables include carrots, parsley, celery, watercress, endive or romaine lettuce, and snap beans. Juice them daily for severe illness and as a foundation of anti-cancer diets. Steamed spinach—an excellent source of vitamins C and A, iron, and potassium—cleanses and reconditions the lymphatic, urinary, and digestive systems. Raw spinach juice is not recommended because its oxalic acid interferes with calcium absorption. All sorts of squash are cleansing and laxative and reduce cholesterol.

Medicinal Mushrooms

Humid weather demands additional cleansing because liver activity is hampered by allergens. Zhu ling (*Polyporus umbellatus*) works as a tumor fighter for lung, bladder, and liver. It enhances immunity. Studies in China have shown it helpful for regaining vitality depleted by chemotherapy and radiation therapy after lung cancer. Zhu Ling is a natural antibiotic, an anti-inflammatory liver protector that is diuretic. It has been proven effective in the treatment of chronic hepatitis B.

If you tend to have urinary tract infections or jaundiced skin, or live and work in a polluted environment, if you have a history of liver disease or habits that damage the liver, or if you travel to unsafe areas, Zhu ling extract is your friend. A good dosage is 40–60 drops of the extract daily.

Summer or Intense Hot Climate
Influence: Heart, small intestine,
and internal temperature
Issues: Odors, ruddy, dry or troubled complexion,
water retention, and overheating

Hot weather makes most people perspire more than normal, which leads to water retention, a puffy face, or heavy legs. To correct this, we increase cleansing foods such as laxative and diuretic green salads. The herbs' cleansing action compensates for our natural weakness resulting from the weather.

Cooling Teas and Beverages

Green Tea Is an All-Around Cleanser and Weight-Loss Tea

One of the best bitter-tasting cleansing stimulants is green tea, which contains less than half the caffeine found in coffee. All teas—white, green, red, oolong, or black—come from the camellia sinensis leaf. The less-processed white and green teas contain the least caffeine, and black tea has the most caffeine. According to recent research, tannins (acids) found in tea reduce cholesterol, protect the elasticity of blood vessels, and detoxify the body. Tea prevents flushed complexion and fragile capillaries better than coffee. Since green tea is laxative and diuretic, it reduces complexion problems and body odors. Summer is a good time to reduce high-calorie and high-fat meals. The following delicious teas will keep you cool, refreshed, and relaxed.

Chinese Chrysanthemum Flower Tea Clears Eye Irritation and Headache

This sweet flower beverage (not a tea leaf) is easy to find in Chinese super-markets or online. Quickly rinse one handful of flowers with a little hot water to remove any dust. Then cover them with boiling water and watch how they open in the glass pitcher. You can serve this tea hot or cold unsweetened. Chrysanthemum flower has a naturally sweet flavor. The tea is recommended by Chinese herbalists to prevent and treat migraine headaches, heat and sun stroke, dizziness, and red swollen eyes. Chrysanthemum flowers can be combined with magnolia buds in a tea to clear sinus congestion. Drink either tea only between meals.

Liquid Chlorophyll and Aloe Drinks Cleanse Your Breath

If you are in a big hurry, here is an instant drink that nourishes the blood as it refreshes your breath and cleanses the entire body. Add 2 tablespoons of health-food store liquid chlorophyll to sparkling water. Drink it anytime to insure internal freshness. If you're constipated, if you get headaches from pollution or perfumes, if you have blemishes, bad breath, and body odor, or if you develop a bad temper before your period, add up to ¼ cup daily of aloe vera gel to water, juice, or tea. Anti-acid aloe reduces nervous hunger. You'll feel and look better.

Cooling Fruits and Vegetables

Hot weather increases sweating and reduces urination. Because of that, acid can build up in the joints or skin and cause a lot of trouble such as acne, eczema, and swollen red joints. Bing cherries and black cherry concentrate reduce uric acid, helping to prevent and treat aching joints and gout. Each morning, add at least 1 tablespoon of the cherry concentrate to water as a liver flush. Also cooling and laxative are pears, apricots, plums, and prunes.

Spring and summer salads should contain several slightly bitter-tasting, cleansing greens such as fiddlehead ferns, watercress, and endive. They will feel cooling and refreshing. Add important minerals to your weight-loss diet with asparagus and okra. Okra is an essential food for anyone who wants to reduce joint swelling and pain. Cabbage, broccoli, and other foods in the cabbage family are known cancer fighters. They increase alkalinity and reduce blemishes and acid conditions such as bad breath, excess hunger, and heartburn. All sprouted seeds and grains contain essential vitamins, minerals, and chlorophyll. I will have more to say about them in later chapters covering slimming, a flawless complexion, and thick hair.

How to Sprout

The simplest way to sprout seeds, beans, or lentils is a method that I use in my Chelsea kitchen, where I am a farmer without a terrain. You should use raw organic seeds such as sunflower or radish or grains—among them lentils, alfalfa, mung or aduki beans, soy beans, wheat berries, or chick peas. Poor-quality seeds will not sprout. I have even sprouted spicy fenugreek (spice) pods. Fenugreek sprouts are recommended to balance blood sugar for diabetes and to improve breathing and energy.

Put ¼ cup of raw seeds, beans, or grains into a wide-mouthed quart jar. Cover the jar with one layer of cheesecloth cut to fit the top and fasten it with a rubber band. The cheesecloth will allow the sprouts to breathe as they grow. Soak the seeds overnight in water that nearly reaches the top of the jar. The seeds will expand. Avoid heat and sun.

The next morning, rinse the seeds with fresh water without removing the cheesecloth. Place the jar sideways in an unlit oven or dark cupboard so that the sprouts can grow. For the next two days rinse the sprouts again once or twice daily until they have grown to the right size, usually about ½ to 1 inch. Sprouts that are too old or long taste bitter. Keep them in the refrigerator until you use them in salads or as a side dish.

Wheat grass, found in many health-food stores, is a concentrated food extremely rich in nutrients and strongly cleansing. I have met people at the beautiful Hippocrates Health Institute in West Palm Beach, Florida, who have learned to live on sprouts and raw foods. Several people I met there had lost from 70 to 100 pounds and looked wonderful. They drink from 1 to 4 ounces daily of fresh wheat-grass juice. It is one of the best sources of vitamin E, an antioxidant and potent rejuvenator. Wheat-grass sprouts are three times higher a source of vitamin E than the seed. According to Ann Wigmore, in *The Sprouting Book*, vitamin E found in sprouted seeds, grains, and nuts such as oats, rye, alfalfa, sesame, sunflower, and almonds, is at least 10 times more easily assimilated than synthetic vitamin E.

Medicinal Mushrooms

Hot climate or inflammatory symptoms such as acne, chronic thirst and dryness, or arthritis require a cooling mushroom such as ling zhi (*Gano-*

derma lucidum) extract. Its anti-tumor, immune-enhancing, anti-viral, and cholesterol-reducing actions are famous. It is considered the "immortality" mushroom by Chinese herbalists. Recent research has found that it increases T cells, natural immune-protector cells. Its benefits have been compared to the drug Prednisone for the treatment of arthritis, except it has no side effects. Ling zhi (a.k.a. reishi) enhances the oxygen-absorbing capacity of the lungs to increase stamina. It is a major HIV drug in Japan and Korea.

Anyone with dull, lifeless skin, shortness of breath, chronic illness and fatigue, or joint aches should add ling zhi to their daily routine. I cook this one regularly in a crockpot and drink it cold like a bitter, slightly foamy mushroom "beer." People who prefer a sweeter flavor can add dried figs, dong quai, or preserved Chinese dates while cooking. For broken facial capillaries, add a handful of sliced raw tienchi ginseng while cooking from 4–6 hours. If you are using ling zhi extract, 40–60 drops are recommended daily.

Indian Summer: Overwork, Poor Digestion, and Jet Lag
Influence: Stomach, spleen, pancreas, and elimination
Issues: Fat, cellulite, puffy skin, bags under eyes, or oozing sores

Most of us battle a sweet tooth or unsightly bulge year round. Bad eating habits weaken digestion and the elimination of impurities. So do late nights, overwork, pollution, and jet lag. Chapter 6, Spot Slimming, contains a basic diet that reduces fat and cholesterol as well as special herbs to reduce problem areas. Poor digestion and fatigue increase water retention. You know you have it if your fingerprint leaves its impression in your flesh. Touch the area near the inside of your ankle to see if the skin bounces back or a dent stays in puffy skin. Water retention in the face makes you look bloated with swollen skin around the eyes. Jet travel is famous for causing water retention. Look at your legs after a few hours of flight. They will look swollen and feel achy.

Mellow, humid weather is relaxing—so is a rich meal followed by a nap. Both slow metabolism. Sweet, creamy, and fried foods produce what Chinese doctors call "internal dampness" (*she*). It refers to mucus congestion and slow metabolism, the underlying problems that can lead to cellulite and fibroids.

Pungent digestive foods and most teas work best during long flights and following celebration feasts. A spicy mint capsule available from East Indian groceries or a cup of hot ginger or green tea will pick up your energy. A snack of green tea and lots of fresh celery helps you avoid the effects of poor digestion and circulation. If possible, take a brisk walk after eating to help work off calories. Eat five small meals daily in order to speed metabolism. One large meal signals the body to store fat during a fast. That slows metabolism to prevent starvation. Then the meal you eat at the end of the day turns to fat. Frequent small slimming meals encourage weight loss.

Slimming, Digestive Beverages

Toasted Barley/Green Tea for a Slimmer Waistline

Digestive foods and diuretic teas reduce water retention in your spare tire. Cooked barley is recommended to prevent water retention. Japanese toasted barley green tea is slimming. You can find it in Japanese groceries and online.

Rejuvelac for Energy, Digestion, and Weight Loss

A fast way to lose extra pounds and water retention is to drink Rejuvelac. One-half cup or more of this mildly pleasant tasting laxative drink before meals washes you clean as it provides valuable nutrients found in sprouts.

Ann Wigmore in *The Sprouting Book* recommends using ½ cup of soft pastry wheat berries and 6 cups of spring or filtered water. Soak winter wheat berries in a half-gallon jar, covered with cheesecloth for 10–15 hours. Drain off the water (do not rinse the wheat berries) and let the wheat sprout for two days. After that, pour water over the wheat sprouts (use about three times the amount of wheat sprouts). Cover the jar and leave it at room temperature for 24 hours. Then pour off the liquid Rejuvelac into another jar. Cover and refrigerate. It keeps for several days. The wheat sprouts can be reused two more times to make additional Rejuvelac. Start by pouring more water over the sprouts and proceed as described. Store Rejuvelac in the refrigerator. Ideally it should be served at room temperature, ½ cup or more before meals.

Chinese Fu-Ling for Bloated Legs

The Chinese herb fu ling (*Poria cocos*) is recommended for water retention, slow or difficult urination, and bloating in the abdomen and legs. Simmer a handful of dried fu ling in 1 quart of water for half an hour and pour it over your favorite tea. Or cook fu ling with grains such as barley or millet (a seed).

Slimming Fruits and Vegetables

Indian summer, because it comes between spring and fall, can use foods from either season. A breakfast of raw vegetables along with hot green tea is especially slimming because it reduces mucus as well as fat. To avoid are sweet root vegetables such as beets and carrots (especially bad for diabetics), which are too high in sugar.

One popular Asian dish used to reduce water retention is barley soup with lotus seeds and dioscurea (Chinese white yam). The latter is a precursor to progesterone that reduces water retention. Dried barley, lotus, and dioscurea soup comes prepackaged in Chinese groceries. Dense seeds such as lotus absorb moisture. Instead of potatoes, I prefer cooking yucca root. It helps joints to slip more smoothly. It cushions joint action and prevents joint swelling. Potatoes contain much more sugar than yucca, especially if you keep them in the refrigerator.

Medicinal Mushrooms

God's Mushroom (*Agaricus blazei*) is called songrong in Chinese. It has exceptionally strong anti-tumor properties as well as interferon and inter-leukin (anti-cancer) effects. It has anti-viral, cholesterol-reducing, and blood-sugar modulating effects. It has been proven effective against Salmonella. Dr. Andrew Weil is particularly enthusiastic about this mushroom and encourages its use in cooking and as a medicine.

The enokitake or enoki (*Flammulina velutipes*) or golden needle mushroom is famous for preventing lung cancer where it is grown in Japan. Studies show that workers within 50 miles of its harvest site suffer much less frequently from cancer. Enoki also offers exciting good results in reducing hypertension. This makes enoki quite useful for people troubled by a rich diet and stagnant lifestyle who are at risk of high blood pressure, diabetes, and excess weight.

Lion's Mane (*Hericium erinaceus*) is called yamabushitake in Japanese. Aside from its immuno-stimulant effects, it treats gastritis and stimulates nerve growth regeneration. In China, this species is commonly prescribed for stomach ailments and for prevention of cancer of the gastrointestinal tract. A group of Japanese researchers in 1994 isolated compounds in yamabushitake that stimulate neurons to regrow, which may make this mushroom valuable in the treatment of Alzheimer's disease. The mushroom has a distinctive seafood-like flavor that makes it a nice addition to fish soups. The recom-mended dosage is 40–60 drops of the extract daily.

Autumn: Dry Climate, Smoke, and Dust
Influence: Lungs, large intestine, and skin
Issues: Breathing, energy, and complexion problems

Traditional Chinese medicine (TCM) considers autumn to be drying. If you smoke or inhale secondary cigarette smoke, you will feel exhausted or catch colds in autumn. If you travel to areas of high smoke or chemical pollution, your health and beauty suffer. Asthma is a common problem affecting much of the world, including tourist destinations. I have used traditional herbal and acupuncture medicine to cure the upper respiratory tract infection I caught while traveling through Asia. In New York, after September 11th, a new sort of asthma from chemical smoke has sprung up. Chinese herbs for a flawless complexion, which we will study later, have proved quite helpful for sinus and skin conditions.

Fatigue and reduced oxygen from shallow breath dulls the skin and makes hair fall out. Lung dryness or inflammation hampers blood production and vitality. Air pollution leads to cough, sore throat, and laryngitis. People who smoke have parched, rough skin, dandruff, and bad breath. Lack of oxygen and increased stress produce anxiety. So there you go: smoke, get nervous; see thinning hair, get more nervous; smoke more, get dry skin; panic, smoke more; and so on.

A number of Chinese herbal moisture tonics ensure healthy blood, bones, muscles, and lovely skin and hair because they allow the body to make and keep its own moisture. Such tonics do much more for your beauty than drinking eight glasses of water daily. Large quantities of water weaken digestion. However, moisturizing tonics enable the body to produce natural fluids in all the right places—your skin, hair, fingernails, and sexual areas. They make you feel and look young and juicy.

Moistening, Soothing Teas and Beverages

American Ginseng Tea Increases Saliva and Reduces Sweet Tooth

American ginseng tea is cooling and refreshing, and also easy to find and make. Often American ginseng comes as an instant tea sold in Chinese grocery stores and supermarkets; just add hot or cold water. American ginseng (*Panax quinquefolium*) is different from Chinese ginseng (*Panax ginseng*). Its properties are moistening and refreshing for delicate internal tissue, especially in the stomach and lungs. It is recommended for diabetes, fevers, thirst, night sweats, dry skin, and weight loss because it cools and refreshes. Many people have told me it also helps to curb a sweet tooth. You can drink it often if you are always thirsty.

Pungent Fruits and Vegetables

Sinus congestion can be a special problem in autumn for people who love sweets, rich foods, dairy products, and alcohol. In contrast, TCM recommends pungent foods including raw and cooked radish, ginger, and the spice cardamon as digestive remedies in order to reduce congestion. You might enjoy radish, celery, and carrots as a weight-loss snack along with a slimming tea.

Pungent foods speed digestion and increase energy. Any supermarket offers a wide variety of them, including watercress, Brussels sprouts, and cabbage.

Watercress is a very alkaline food that is effective for weight loss. It helps to purify the body because it is high in vitamins such as A that reduce catarrh. Watercress improves glandular secretions and is high in sulfur and potassium, which makes it a major fat melter.

Brussels sprouts, cabbage, and cauliflower are in the same family. They produce gas for people with weak digestion. To avoid problems, do not eat them with fruit, starch, or beer. Steam them adding caraway seeds and oil after they are cooked. Cabbage is particularly high in vitamins A and B1 and contains many minerals. It is a good source of calcium, potassium, and sulfur, which beautify complexion. Sauerkraut juice, with a little lemon juice added, is helpful for diabetes, sluggish digestion, constipation, bad breath, and especially skin blemishes.

Potatoes can irritate digestion. They are also fattening when stored in the refrigerator. Nourishing, slimming potato substitutes include chayote, beans, and legumes. Chayote contains potassium, magnesium, and silicon. Beans and legumes are good sources of protein and carbohydrates. Lima beans contain potassium, phosphorus, calcium, and iron that increase muscle tone. String beans contain manganese and nitrogen, which improve complexion.

Beet greens contain potassium, magnesium, iodine, and iron to help cleanse and build blood for a radiant glowing complexion. Chervil, eaten in salads or with vegetables, protein, or carbohydrates, replenishes minerals for hair, skin, and nails. Chicory is a bitter cleanser that clears complexion problems and provides iron, sulfur, and potassium. Chives are hot stuff for catarrh. Added to salad or vegetables, chives speed elimination of fats with potassium, calcium, and sulfur. Limit their use if you have stomach ulcers or urinary problems.

If you have a dry cough, thirst, and lizard dry skin, add cooked oatmeal and asparagus to your daily menu.

Medicinal Mushrooms

Cordyceps sinensis (dong chong xia cao) reduces just about any type of stress. Chinese cooks add it to chicken and duck soup for its pleasant bitter, salty flavoring. Since it relaxes bronchials and deepens respiration, it increases oxygen uptake and reduces blemishes, infections, and fatigue.

Shiitake (*Lentinula edodes*) or, in Chinese, xiang gu, is recommended anytime as a delicious dish. Its natural disease-killer action and interferon make it a powerful immune booster. It fortifies the liver against stress and poisons. It has been used as an injectable anti-cancer drug in Asia. It reduces cholesterol and is anti-viral. An extract from shiitake has been shown effective against type 1 herpes simplex virus. This mushroom has also been suggested for the treatment of chronic fatigue syndrome. It is relatively inexpensive compared to many other mushroom species. You can buy it dried in China-towns around the world and cook it with soup or stir-fried vegetables. The rec-ommended dosage for the extract is 40–60 drops daily.

Winter or Cold, Harsh Climate
Influence: Kidneys, adrenal glands, and hormones
Issues: Vitality, sexuality, enthusiasm, dull or gray skin hue, and dark circles around the eyes

Winter's cold blustery weather can drain vitality, especially if you are tired and stressed from work or emotional upset. You may want to stay under the covers during this season. You may put on a few pounds from eating richly and sleeping more than usual. To avoid excess weight gain, add a few energy tonic herbs to speed metabolism and lift vitality and enthusiasm. Cold and damp weather, jet lag, overwork, illness, or stimulants such as coffee and black tea challenge adrenal energy. You may feel and look pale and lethargic. Herbal tonics that increase stamina and immunity are often warming and stim-ulating in quality.

Winter is the time to stress energy tonics and adaptogens such as the gin-sengs. The holidays are a great time to socialize and you will want to look and feel your best. It is a time to have romantic breakfasts in bed. You will want sexual energy and drive to be up to speed.

Spicy, Stimulating Teas and Beverages

A pinch of one of the following herbs in a mug of hot water, when steeped for a few minutes, will give you a bracing energy pickup. Sage, rosemary, thyme, and cinnamon brighten complexion. Unless you feel feverish or have hot flashes, you can use these teas to increase energy, deepen breath, and build immunity to cold weather's draining effects. Sage is a general stimulant, a Western equivalent to Chinese ginseng. It prevents chills, fatigue, and excess sweating from weakness. Use it when tired and when skin sags from fatigue. Rosemary is a strong stimulant to adrenal and heart energy. Be careful to use only a small pinch when cooking or making this tea. Otherwise, you may experience temporary heart irregularities. It warms the complexion to counter pallor and sallow complexion. Thyme is a stimulant for breathing that is recommended for wheezing asthma. As a beauty beverage, use it for dull, oxygen-starved skin.

Cinnamon tea facilitates sweating and stimulates blood circulation, which is a fine way to prevent aches from a cold or hypothermia. Add up to ⅛ teaspoon to hot water as a tea between meals to bring color to your face. If you have blemishes, avoid cinnamon and all other hot spices.

Supportive Fruits and Vegetables for Minerals and Energy

A high-stress lifestyle or a cold climate are good reasons to increase rich, nourishing foods such as almonds and apricots. They make a complexion-beautifying snack. Avocado is full of helpful oils and vitamins for the skin. Root vegetables such as carrots, parsnips, turnips, and turnip leaves improve eye health.

Black currents, dried dates, black figs, peaches, pears, persimmons, pineapple, pomegranate, or walnuts make nourishing non-fattening desserts. Sweet warming spices such as clove, cinnamon, allspice, and cardamom can be strong stimulants. Use them wisely one pinch at a time. For example, peaches made with a dash of spicy clove powder are a strong stimulant for breathing as well as an aphrodisiac for tired lovers. However, people who experience fever, hypertension, or hot flashes may become dizzy or get a headache. Oranges are acidic and hard to digest. Avoid them if you have complexion blemishes.

Chinese Tonic Soup Stocks For Complexion Beauty

Chinese tonic herbs, used to strengthen internal organs, also improve complexion by enhancing blood production and circulation. Some can be added to flavor and fortify soups. A basic soup stock can be made from simmering any herb or food in water for about one hour. Strain the liquid, which becomes the soup stock. You can either reuse the herb or not as you prefer. When cooking expensive or tasty herbs, I reuse them a second time with new water and eat the tasty ones.

For example, I add one piece each of dong quai and Chinese ginseng, both warming stimulants, to my soups in order to prevent weakness at any season. Cooking tonic herbs such as these helps with digestion of the soup ingredients and costs less than taking pep pills. If your family tends to have high cholesterol and high blood pressure, you ought to substitute cooling raw tienchi ginseng for the above herbs. Raw tienchi ginseng increases circulation, reduces bruising, and prevents internal bleeding, while it reduces cholesterol and chest pains. If your complexion is too ruddy or if you bruise easily, add ¼ teaspoon of raw tienchi ginseng powder to a little water as a tea twice daily until inflammation cools. Or cook sliced raw tienchi in a soup stock.

Medicinal Mushrooms

Paul Stamets (www.fungi.com) makes a combination extract using seven top quality medicinal mushrooms. I recommend it for anyone especially concerned with maintaining vitality and beauty. Stamets 7 Mushroom Blend contains royal sun agaricus, cordyceps, reishi (ling zhi), maitake, lion's mane, zhu ling, and yun zhi. Using the combination between meals for a total of 40–60 drops daily gives full-spectrum protection found in these medicinal treasures.

Staying well and beautiful is a matter of staying in harmony with the weather or the seasons and overcoming your particular energy weaknesses. Following the above guide will help you to avoid stress.

A Quick Fix to Clear Your Senses

Discomfort	Quick Food Remedy
Slow digestion, sinus congestion	Radish
Red eyes, thirst, hot weather	Chrysanthemum flower tea
Thirst, dry mouth, fatigue	American ginseng tea

Especially for Men

Both men and women now take "extreme" vacations. A new industry has grown to service people who *want* to risk their lives for fun. Once a Hungarian friend and former director of the New York Explorer's Club told me about his vacation to Antarctica, where he was followed for several days by a polar bear! He prepared for his ice trek by eating extra-fat beef for a month before leaving in order to "thicken his blood."

You can thicken or pollute your blood during a business meeting or a night out and still keep your youthful figure and nice complexion by adding lecithin, omega 3 and 6 fish oils, or flax seed oil to your daily routine. They protect your cholesterol level. A daily dose of 500–1000 mg of niacinamide (vitamin B_3) is thought to reduce high triglycerides.

Drinking aloe vera gel (which you can mix in apple juice) after excess eating and drinking can prevent heartburn. Taking a big dose of B vitamins before you go out drinking will reduce your chances of a hangover. Homeopathic nux vomica 30C taken between meals is recommended for sinus congestion and hangover pain. It also helps for chronic migraines or crabbiness from too much work, worry, and medication.

Lola's Way

The culture we enjoy and memories we make while traveling remain forever. Don't let travel fatigue and illness mar your trip. When flying, you should use herbs and foods to maintain normal digestion and circulation. A flight from New York to Hong Kong can take nearly 20 hours under normal circumstances. After you arrive, the room may spin from your fatigue or inner-ear problems. I take a capsule of valerian (*Valeriana officinalis*), a nerve relaxer, every several hours or as needed during a flight to reduce dizziness, migraine headache, and in-flight insomnia. In Chapter 14, I will share advice from a leading beauty expert on how to arrive without looking tired and puffy.

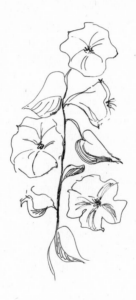

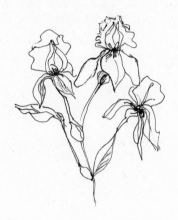

PART TWO

Your New Body

What you notice about someone walking toward you are
the energy in the step, the person's shape, and how these
things encompass their being.

5

Your Walk

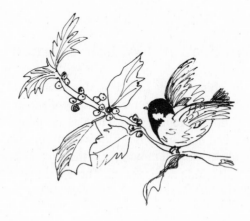

One who loves beauty enhances life each moment.

One evening on Miami beach, we sat at an open-air café in balmy weather as people strolled hand in hand listening to a band play. One young couple caught my attention. He walked straight ahead, intent on getting somewhere. His companion had a slim, supple body that might have been beautiful except that she crept like a dog following a master. I couldn't tell whether she lacked confidence or was in pain.

Your walk reveals your sense of self. The space taken by your easy stride indicates your comfort zone and limits. Your walk is an important means of communication. Moving merely to get somewhere, you miss the benefits that come from flirting. Imagine the number of beautifying hormones and endorphins (natural pain-killers) necessary to make you look and feel sexy? Your graceful walk can give you and others a pleasing energy boost. Vitality is created moment to moment for the person in touch with his or her body. Accept your beauty as a gift to share: imagine yourself tall and relaxed as you walk so that you move with assurance. Your poise signals to others how you wish to be treated.

My New York walk has a quick, no-nonsense step that does not invite conversation with strangers. It is shaped by muscles that support my frame. You can make yourself look fat or thin, weak or strong, tired or sexy with your walk. It depends on where you place your center of gravity. One woman I observed was petite but with each step she seemed to grow fatter in the hips. She collapsed her center of gravity and clomped along with heavy feet—all you saw were her hips. Following are daily exercises and teas that improve balance and ease of movement, the physical and energetic basis of a healthy, alluring walk.

A Beautiful Walk Is Learned

I asked a few of my chiropractor friends to describe a healthy walk. Dr. Vittoria Repetto, who practices chiropractic and applied kinesiology in downtown New York, said, "A beautiful walk moves smoothly without stopping, jarring, or jerking. The heel hits first, followed by the flat of the foot, with weight on the outside of the ball moving into the center of the ball of the foot, then the push off—all in one even motion. There is an even swing of legs and arms as you walk."

Alignment

Aligning the posture is like building a house: you have to start with a good foundation. Proper posture is centered with your spine leaning neither too far forward nor too far backward. Your center of gravity should be in your pelvis. You have seen good alignment before if, as a child, you had an inflatable toy clown. This clown has a wide, rounded bottom, so that it bounces back to an upright position when punched.

You can observe your alignment by standing sideways in front of a full-length mirror. Look at an object some distance in front of you. Then turn only your head to observe your side view in the mirror. Are you leaning forward to see the object? If so, your walk may look as though your are straining and hurried. Are you leaning backward as though afraid to move? Are you sway-backed? These may indicate problems with balance or the placement of your weight on to your feet.

Backache Home Remedies

Many alignment problems can be improved with remedies for chronic back pain. For example, you may enjoy an afternoon cup of hot nettle or damiana tea in order to improve adrenal vitality. A strong back will help you stand straighter. Homeopathic magnesium phosphate 6x added to water reduces spasms and tight muscle discomforts in the entire body.

According to a number of western doctors I have interviewed, vitamin D and magnesium deficiencies are epidemic in America. "Trying to avoid sun damage, we end up with weak bones and tense muscles," was one comment. Vitamin D is not a problem for many Asians. Not only do they believe in walking in the sun, they eat freshwater and saltwater eel, nature's highest natural source of vitamin D. In Japan, a special August festival is devoted to celebrating the summer with eel dishes, which are considered strengthening.

Dr. Marcey Shapiro, a beautiful herbalist and acupuncturist as well as Western-trained medical doctor from the Berkeley area, recommends high doses of St. John's wort, at least 500 mg three times daily, in order to prevent chronic backache. Her association with herbs is sensitive and personalized. She believes you have to communicate with herbs, trees, and flowers to enjoy their full benefit. An earth goddess at heart, her garden overflows with thyme, sage, and 4-foot-high artichoke plants. Her easy graceful walk comes from respect for nature, a dignified and loving association with plants. She looks as though she could be at ease anywhere because her feet are firmly planted on the earth.

An Exercise Especially for Your Spine

To help straighten your walk, you might also try this exercise: lift your spine, neck, and head gently up toward the ceiling, while stretching your legs tall and spreading your toes. That stretches you in both directions toward the ceiling and floor. Imagine that you are a Grecian pillar—rooted in the earth while touching the sky. Take a few steps forward. Your pelvis should move up and down no more than 2 inches. The pelvis shifts from side to side as you walk but should not oscillate more than 1 inch. You may have to practice your walk in front of a mirror or with someone watching to avoid bobbing up and down, shifting back and forth like a washing machine agitator, or swaying too far off balance.

The Daily Prayer Position and Your Posture

Chiropractor Rita Ghiraldini, a Brazilian-born beauty, complains, "Some girls walk like football players! No matter how I feel about equal rights, this is absolutely ridiculous! Who wants to look like a primate?" She thinks that walking as though balancing a book on your head has good effects. She says, "While sitting, have the head balanced above the tail bone, with feet shoulder length apart and both feet flat touching the ground. That brings everything into perfect alignment on the inside." Here is a daily exercise that Rita does five to ten times daily to improve posture:

1. Put palms together at the heart with fingers pointing upward as if praying.
2. Bring elbows out to the sides with the forearms parallel to the floor.
3. Relax the shoulder blades down and toward one another in the back.
4. Hold for a couple of seconds and release.

Rita considers poor alignment to be a major cause of scoliosis (abnormally curved spine). She says, "faulty arches don't support the person's weight properly, then the pelvis drops on one side, and creates the scoliosis." To get into the mood, you might do the prayer position while inhaling deeply and listening to soothing music.

Exercise/Massage for Your Arches

Your arches are the basis of a balanced walk and consistent muscle strength in your legs. One fantastic Flamenco dancer who has a stage career into her sixties suggested an exercise to develop flexible, strong arches. Standing barefoot, pick up a handkerchief or marbles with your toes. I suggest massaging your arches with Epsom salts in a hot bath. Make sure to press and move in a circular motion at the center of your arch. It is on the bottom of each foot where the ball changes from darker to lighter-colored flesh. That area contains acupuncture points important for arthritis, leg pain, and water retention in the legs.

Stretches for Chronic Back and Leg Pain

Many of us sit trapped at computers or workstations all day long. We stretch infrequently or walk in high heels, which tilt the pelvis forward. Because of this, the lumbar vertebrae (at the lower back) are crunched together creating stiffness and pain. My beautiful cats would never do such a foolish thing. See how they stretch first thing in the morning.

Right now, jump off your seat like a cat onto all fours—balancing your weight on the palms of your hands and your knees. Gently tuck in your hips toward your chest. Pull your spine up into a convex curve toward the ceiling. Then reverse: dip your spine gently down into a concave curve so that shoulders and behind are higher. That gentle spinal stretch, known as the cat posture in yoga, can help to keep your vertebrae "well-oiled."

If you wear high heels, the ligaments behind your knees will suffer pain and tightness. Make sure to stretch them out every evening in this way: stand barefoot in a doorway or on a book so that the balls of your feet are 2 inches higher than your heels. Feel the stretch behind your legs. To continue the stretch, lift your spine up from the pelvis to your head. Reach with arms to the ceiling, then bend over gently as though you could touch the floor with your hands.

Nutrition and Herbs

Proper nutrition and herbs help centering and balance because they build strength. Rita Ghiraldini recommends calcium carbonate for all women (1200–1500 mg per day). She believes that "milk doesn't do the job." One of my favorite herbal sources of calcium carbonate is Chinese pearl powder. The advantage of using pearl powder is that it calms the nerves while it provides calcium. The recommended dose is the contents of one small glass tube (approximately ⅛ teaspoon) of pearl powder poured into a little water and taken before bed.

For a calm, confident walk, I cook at low heat overnight in a crockpot one tube of pearl powder along with one handful each of several blood-enhancing herbs. I normally use *Rehmannia glutinosa* (shu di huang) and *Cistanches herba* (rou cong rong) along with 4 cups of water. If the weather is cold or I feel weak, I may add one piece of *Angelica sinensis* (dong quai) in order to improve my circulation. The recommended dosage of the semi-sweet brew is 1–3 cups between meals. Rehmannia and cistanches are moistening and laxative if used to excess.

Supplements that increase the natural shock-absorbers between joints reduce pain and swelling. Rita recommends glucosamine sulfate for cartilage regeneration especially for women after age 30 or younger if there is a family history of juvenile rheumatoid arthritis or lupus.

One of my favorite food sources of joint protection is yucca, which can be prepared like boiled potato and seasoned with garlic and vinegar. Sea cucumber, an ugly water creature that swims the shallow waters off China and Japan, is made into soups and dishes valued in the East for their tonic properties. Sea cucumber, which is also recommended for preventing joint damage, is sometimes found in Chinese restaurants and takes hours of soaking and cooking. For the less courageous, Health Concerns makes Sea-Q (sea cucumber dietary supplement pills). See the Annotated Resource Guide for more details.

Those powerful vitality-enriching herbs can help you to attain a measure of emotional security. If you feel rooted in your body—relaxed and strong deep down to your bone marrow—your walk will not sway, wobble, or creep.

With one foot firmly planted in front of the other, you can spread your webs like a duck and softly tread past mud puddles and tight spots in your life.

Fatigue, Back Pain, and Adrenal Weakness

If you have chronic back pain, every step will be miserable. Traditional Chinese herbalists believe that exhaustion, poor dietary habits, cold weather, and long hours sitting or standing can reduce vital energy. They believe it can eventually lead to lower back and knee pain, urinary incontinence, sexual weakness, and even impairment of hearing and eyesight.

Certain Chinese herbal supplements are formulated to reverse the signs of exhaustion and chronic back pain. Many contain stimulants that Chinese herbalists call warming herbs. These make muscles feel stronger and warmer, while they increase energy and circulation. However, warming, stimulating herbal combinations should not be used when symptoms of inflammation are present, such as fever, chronic thirst, rapid pulse or heartbeat, painful or diminished urination, insomnia, dry eyes, constipation, or irritability.

Backbone (Bu Shen Huo Xue Dietary Supplement) is a warming pill remedy for back pain that is made by Health Concerns. Backbone's formula contains the following herbs: eucommia, psoralea, cibotium, cuscuta, cistanche, rehmannia, gui ban, cyathula, acanthopanax, tang kuei tips, dipsacus, carthamus, myrrh, and cornus. The pills are recommended if lower back pain is accompanied by weakness, chronic chills, frequent clear urination, or sexual weakness. Several of its ingredients, such as cuscuta, cornus, and eucommia, naturally stimulate testosterone. The formula stimulates adrenal energy and strongly increases circulation in the lower back and legs.

The herbal pills, swallowed between meals, might feel like a warming back massage. The formula can be used in order to increase muscle strength. It may also help the body to maintain chiropractic adjustments longer (as long as inflammation symptoms do not occur). The recommended dose for men or women is 3 tablets three times daily between meals. Discontinue use if the above signs of inflammation occur.

Varicose Veins

Last season, I was the herbalist for a professional indoor soccer team. It was nice having handsome clients with great legs. One player had chronic varicose veins that had nothing to do with exercise but indicated poor circulation and poor calcium absorption.

Herbs that tone blood vessels and increase circulation are often recommended for varicose veins or tired legs. One combination made by Futurebi-otics is called Leg-Aid, and is sold as a "support supplement for leg muscles and veins." Leg-Aid contains niacin to increase circulation; MSM, a form of sulphur that reduces inflammatory pain and waste from the body; citrus bioflavonoids to firm blood vessels; glucosamine sulfate to reduce joint pains; and grapeseed extract, horse chestnut, butcher's broom, prickly ash bark, and ginkgo to tone circulation.

The recommended dose of 2 pills daily may not be enough to help long-term serious varicose veins and pain. The combination is very healthful and safe, but long-time use may be necessary before you can see and feel results.

The best homeopathic remedy for varicose veins is homeopathic calc. fluor. 6x (calcium fluoride), which tones all weak internal organs and improves a variety of circulation problems. If you want to improve your circulation on a daily basis, you might add up to 10 pills of homeopathic calc. fluor. 6x to 1 quart of spring water and drink it as you walk to work or exercise at the gym.

The Turnout

The turnout is done by pointing your toes diagonally from your body instead of straight in front of you. Although highly prized in ballet, it is unnatural for your walk and eventually damages the legs, tendons, and hip joints. Many people do it without trying because one leg is shorter or more tense than the other. Eventually the strain placed on one leg can increase joint size and lead to arthritic discomfort. It may eventually affect balance, alignment, and back pain.

Corrective shoes are not always the answer. Sometimes your posture has compensated for so long that adding a lift in your shoe may cause further pain or damage to the spine. Whenever possible, it is better to strengthen weak muscles. According to TCM, muscles can spasm because of overstimulation or poor circulation affecting an acupuncture meridian. In the case of the turnout or sciatica (pain along the sciatic nerve), circulation is trapped in the Chinese acupuncture meridian that is related to the gallbladder. It runs down the outside of each leg to the outside of the foot. The inner leg muscles (and meridians) can also become weak.

An Exercise

Many dancers practice until their feet bleed, but you don't need to. Here is an easy exercise you can practice at home to relieve pain and correct a turnout.

Stand relaxed and balanced with your feet shoulder-width apart and point-ing straight in front of you. Take a few breaths into the lower abdomen and let the air fall to the ground, traveling down through your legs. At the same time, lift upward gently with your spine, neck, and head in order to stretch and relax the spine.

Find a line on the sidewalk and follow the line, walking with one foot in front of the other on the line. You may have to think of turning your toes inward toward each other in order to straighten your feet. This walk keeps you from pointing your feet outward like Charlie Chaplin's famous waddle. Another suggestion for a smooth, pain-free walk is Mobility 2 herbal pills made by Health Concerns. The formula treats chronic inflammation and poor circulation affecting the muscles and joints. The pills reduce burning pain from gout, sciatica, and lumbago as well as correct underlying problems such as edema (water retention). Its Chinese herbal ingredients enhance blood cir-culation to ease movement.

Weak Leg Muscles

Does fatigue make every step an effort? Do you bump into furniture or drop things from your hands when you are tired? Aswagandha is the East Indian name for a form of ginseng, which works particularly well for strengthening muscles and the lower back. It is recommended as an energy tonic for athlet-ics as well as for pregnancy. Women need strong back muscles and lots of endurance in order to push during delivery.

Aswagandha reduces fatigue while it protects the nerves. I have recom-mended it for people so weak that they could not get out of bed. It makes them feel stronger and reduces nervous anxiety and exhaustion insomnia. You can find aswagandha powder and capsules in East Indian groceries in New York and in many health-food stores.

You can safely use it if you have a pale tongue and chronic weakness or chills. I add ¼ teaspoon of ashwagandha powder to hot water as a tea to brace my energy and enthusiasm during cold weather. *Codonopsis,* a neutral gin-seng called dang shen in Chinese, is recommended for prolapse problems such as chronic diarrhea and hemorrhoids resulting from weakness. Because it lifts energy and tones metabolism, it may be helpful for tired legs.

Prevent Injury and Speed Healing

Runners, athletes, models, and people who sit or stand for long hours need a steady source of vitamins and minerals such as those found in bee pollen and

Chinese Royal Jelly. They make a sweet treat that won't endanger your waist-line. If you have back or leg pain from a sprain or injury, take this tip recom-mended by most chiropractors: eat a handful of papaya enzyme (papain) pills or pineapple enzyme (bromelain) pills several times daily in order to reduce inflammatory wastes from the bloodstream. It will speed healing.

Here are two easy stretches that can help to prevent back pain and injury from overexertion. For 5 minutes daily, stand like a tall, green tree to feel rooted and do the following exercise: with bare feet firmly planted shoulder-width apart, reach with arms to the ceiling. Hold to a count of five, release, and relax. Repeat and gradually increase the count to 10. Make wide, gentle counterclockwise circles with all your moving joints, starting from your head until you reach your toes.

How to Improve Your Walk

At breakfast, add a pinch of turmeric powder to your tea to improve overall circulation. For the rest of the day, relax tight tendons with several doses of homeopathic ruta grav. 30C taken between meals. It is easiest to dissolve 10 pills in a container of water and sip it. At night, soak feet for 10 minutes in hot water and Epsom salts. Then massage feet and legs with your favorite lotion. Circulation and muscle tone can improve if you massage according to the natural flow of acupuncture meridians: move strokes upward on the inside (ventral) side of the legs and downward on the outside (lateral) side.

To improve circulation, I use an anti-cellulite cream called Spanish Gar-den Body Slimming Cream made by VS Labs USA in Beverly Hills. Its ingre-dients include aloe vera gel, ivy extract, and extracts of papain, ginseng, calendula, ascophyllum, and collagen. Another leg slimming cream from Chi-natown is called Sweeten and contains seaweed, diuretic poria (fu ling), angelica, and ginger. When massaged into chubby thighs for 10 minutes twice daily it is said to catabolize surplus fat within six weeks and give wonderful results in three months.

For a course in coordination and grace, watch some movies from Holly-wood's Golden Age. How do Rita Hayworth, Lauren Bacall, and Katherine Hepburn walk? Their center of gravity looks lower than our modern, head-long lunge. They hurry with grace and assurance. Greer Garson once said, "My walk is described as a floating cathedral." How do Kirk Douglas, Burt Lancaster, Paul Newman, Steve McQueen, or your favorite actor walk? Burt Lancaster had a great physique from being a circus performer. Steve McQueen was light on his feet like a cat. His coordination may have helped him to dodge race cars. What impression does your favorite actor make with his or her walk?

Especially for Men

Surprisingly, I sometimes recommend an herbal sexual tonic for men who complain of backache, tired legs, and poor posture. Energy is necessary for a confident walk! Herbs traditionally recommended for male virility also strengthen back muscles and improve posture and endurance. However, the herbs may be too warming and stimulating for some people.

Unless they have fever, night sweats, insomnia, or irritability, most men can take 1–3 tablets, three times daily, of a typical vitality tonic such as Chinese ginseng or damiana.

I do not recommend yohimbe or guarana, herbs sometimes used for sexual impotence, because they are too irritating and overstimulating. Yohimbe must never be combined with psychological medicines, street drugs, or alcohol because it augments emotional upset. Guarana is an irritating heavy dose of caffeine. I prefer a well-rounded virility tonic that combines herbs for building tissue and fluids as well as sexual drive and power—for example, Virility Tabs made by Health Concerns.

Lola's Way

Lola Montez wrote in *The Arts of Beauty,* "An indistinct, shuffling, irregular, sluggish, and slovenly walk is a tolerably sure sign of corresponding attributes of the soul. And, on the other hand, an affected, pert, wan, and pedantic step draws upon a woman the worst impressions from the opposite gender. But there is a remarkable charm in a walk characterized by blended *dignity and vivacity.* It leaves upon the beholder a lasting impression of those attributes of mind which most surely awaken esteem and admiration."

Dignity and vivacity might be translated here as centering or balance. Your walk shows people who you are and what you want from them and yourself. Plato wrote in his *Symposium,* "Our most intimate need is to prolong and stabilize our good and what we essentially are." How balanced and centered are you? Let's find out by practicing a simple exercise.

While walking alone in the city or country, inhale to a count of six; hold in your breath again counting to six while relaxing; then exhale again for a count of six. Gradually lengthen your count of inhalation, holding, and exhalation up to 12. Try to keep the pace steady. Eventually, you will be able to let your mind wander instead of counting.

- Observe what you see around you.
- Observe how you feel as you pass people and places.
- Observe how people regard you.

The essential you is the part that does not change despite stress, blame, or praise. Your walk is an extension of the peace you find within.

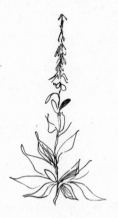

6

Spot Slimming

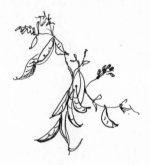

See spot . . . See spot spread . . . See spot go out of control.

Most fitness experts believe that the only way to lose weight is from global fat reduction. A number of fashion models and dancers who are my clients disagree. Spot slimming is a well-kept secret among professionals paid to show their curves. We have developed a safe, effective method that works within two days to one month depending on individual vitality. First, enhance metabolism with a fat-slimming, energy-building diet. In this chapter, several diet options are described in terms of broader beauty-related issues. Then add super-slimming techniques for problem areas. If you are pregnant, avoid all laxative herbs and the slimming massage in this chapter.

America's Fat and Sugar Binge

The fat epidemic, though not on the official agenda, is always a hot topic for participants attending the annual conference on "Botanical Medicine in Modern Clinical Practice" held at Columbia University's medical school. The conference draws health professionals who are enthusiastic to share research information about herbs. I lead walking tours of herb shops in New York's Chinatown and East Indian neighborhoods.

Last May, as we sipped green tea in one of Chinatown's new chic tea parlors, Rita Miller-Huey, a nutritionist prominent in the health industry and co-author of the delightful *43 Ways to Keep You and Your Taste Buddies Happy,* told me, "Americans are getting more sickly and expensive to care for. There is an ever-increasing rate of obesity and diabetes among the young in this country." We all know it: working long hours and eating on the run, digestion becomes sluggish. To satisfy stimulation-hunger, we reach for comfort foods. Stress and fatigue underlie most food addictions because our body craves to maintain homeostasis, even in sickness. We need healthy ways to curb excessive sugar cravings.

Cinnamon for Your Sweet Tooth

Dr. Bud Dansby, a tall, gray-haired, and youthful cardiologist from Fort Myers, Florida, has said, "A diabetic craves sugar when insulin uptake is low." To curb a sweet tooth, cinnamon or fenugreek tea facilitate insulin uptake. Not everyone is diabetic, but many doctors agree we can curb a sugar addiction by strengthening the pancreas. Barring allergies or excess inflammation, you can add up to ¼ teaspoon of cinnamon powder daily to a cup of coffee, tea, or oatmeal

Bud Dansby also recommends vitamins C and E, Coenzyme Q 10 (ubiquinone), and healthy oils such as omega 3 fish oils, flax seed, and evening primrose oil for his patients in order to protect heart health and energy. He knows that enhanced energy leads to good eating habits and improvements in lifestyle. An artist, Bud also recommends oil painting to reduce stress and, as he says, to explore the inner self.

Fats and Sweets for Slimming

Dr. Andrew Weil is one of the star attractions at the conference on botanical medicine. His cogent research information and cheery disposition are a plus. He recommends omega 3 and 6 fish oils found in salmon, tuna, sardines, and mackerel to reduce cholesterol. He eats salmon three times a week along with generous amounts of cholesterol-reducing foods, especially walnuts, walnut oil, and ground fresh flax seeds added to cereal. He says that healthy fats are easily absorbed and eliminated by the body, so they can replace unhealthy fats like butter and margarine. Vegetable fats from beans and avocados are less harmful than dairy products. Artichokes and yucca are good low-fat substitutes for potatoes. For desert, fruit sugars found in apple, pineapple, and papaya are far more slimming than pastry and white bread.

Not all sweets are bad for you. Actually, *Stevia rebaudiana,* a shrub indigenous to South America, is useful for diabetes and has become a popular sugar substitute. Chocolate contains catechins (specialized acids), which help protect the body from cancer and heart disease. Unsweetened baker's chocolate is a high-energy, low-fat pleasure food that contains no cholesterol or sodium, 7 grams of fat, and 70 calories per serving. Beware—chocolate's *caffeine* is addictive.

Make Wellness a Habit

By now, most people know that eating fruits and vegetables reduces the risk of heart trouble. Nevertheless, they cannot always *apply* that sound advice. You can take advantage of the body's tendency to maintain a habit. If energy and digestion feel in balance, you will be less likely to reach for comfort foods. For that, I recommend using homeopathic nux vomica 30C, often recommended for hangover, upset stomach, and moodiness from overeating and drinking, as a regular remedy to encourage a positive attitude and good eating habits. Take one dose (5 pills) between meals three to five times daily to get your body used to craving healthier foods. In other words, treat the problem of addiction in order to avoid it.

Dieting Options and Your Beauty

Getting adequate protein, necessary for healthy bones, muscles, skin, hair, teeth, and every aspect of physical beauty, is a challenge we all face. In March 2000, the Department of Agriculture sponsored a congressional debate between diet book authors situated in two camps—the high-protein, high-fat diet versus the low-protein, fruit, vegetables, and carbohydrate diet—over the ideal weight-loss solution. Highly charged battle lines were drawn between a cardiologist (Robert Atkins), an internist (Dean Ornish), a biochemist (Barry Sears), and a cardiac surgeon (Morrison Bethea). You wonder if any of them can cook worth a darn.

The "hog-wild" high-fat, high-protein group, led by Atkins, believes everyone should eat all meats, including fat ones such as bacon, lamb, shrimp, and duck; eat cream and most cheeses; and reduce daily carbohydrates to 20 grams or one tossed green salad daily. Fruit, bread, grains, starchy vegetables, and skim milk are to be avoided. The "yogi diet" fruit and veggie group, headed by Ornish, recommends heart-saving proteins made up of beans and legumes, as well as fruits, vegetables, and grains. To be avoided are all the meats in Atkins' list as well as fish, chicken, oils, dairy products, sugar, alcohol, and any processed products that contain more than 2 grams of fat per serving.

The well-publicized flap brought to life the nursery rhyme—Jack Sprat could eat no fat and his wife could eat no lean. Which one is right? It pays to look the two options directly in the eye . . . and the waistline. Is there any advantage in loading the body with protein for a couch-potato lifestyle? How do you really want to look, smell, or sound? There is more to dieting than meets the mouth.

To Beef or Not to Beef

Aside from the risk of mad cow disease, the beef and bacon diet can cause beauty problems stemming from the side effects of animal-protein consumption. They include allergies, excess acid reflux, and blemishes from impurities. Meat eaters can easily become hot-tempered folks with inflammatory problems, including body odor, liver spots, and itchy rash. Why? By eating meat we ingest the animal's uric acid, hormones, chemical additives, and intense "slaughter anxiety." That excess inflammation can affect the complexion. In fact, depriving the body of carbohydrates naturally leads to an acid condition called ketosis. As the body draws upon fat as fuel, weight loss follows. However, ketosis withers muscles and waste nerves, especially for those with high-stress lifestyles. Ketosis leads to halitosis and mood swings as the body essentially digests itself. Dr. Andrew Weil has said, "High fat and high protein foods tend to crowd out protective nutrients, including minerals found in fruits and vegetables."

Spend time with heavy animal-protein eaters and you may notice red blemishes, blood-shot eyes, thinning hair, and dark circles under their eyes, indicating multiple allergies and a weakened immune system. Heavy animal-protein eaters have been known to develop chronic fatigue and poor digestion at the same time as gout and high cholesterol. Pain from gout makes people cranky (as seen in Lionel Barrymore movies)! Research is currently underway at the University of Texas Southwestern Medical Center in Dallas to see if the high-protein, low-carbohydrate diet increases the risk of kidney stones and bone loss. Drs. Shalini Reddy and Chia-Ying Wang, both assistant professors of internal medicine, anticipate a thumbs down for high-protein diets.

Clean Protein Alternatives

No one thinks hot flashes or arthritis are attractive. A few researchers are paying close attention to foods that reduce fat and cholesterol as well as keep you younger.

Super Soy: One Block of Tofu Supplies the Day's Calcium and Protein

Alternative medicine doctors have said that soy proteins from cooked soy beans, fresh green soy beans in the pod, and tofu can substitute for animal proteins. Tempeh, fermented soy bean paste, and soy drinks, have the added advantage of helping to balance estrogen production.

Dr. Adriane Fugh-Berman, assistant clinical professor of health care sciences at George Washington University's School of Medicine in Washington, D.C., has researched the effects of soy on women's health. Dr. Fugh-Berman has found breast cancer rates to be significantly lower in China, Korea, and Japan, and links her findings to increased intake of soy, flax seeds, red clover, and sprouts. Dr. Fugh-Berman said that populations whose diets are made up of 47% soy experience lower LDL cholesterol and triglycerides. In one three-year study, post-menopausal women experienced less spinal bone loss because of soy.

The good news is that genistein, the main active ingredient that we look for in soy, is also found in yellow split peas, black beans, baby lima beans, anasazi, and red kidney beans. Other sources include miso (roasted soy beans). The highest calcium content comes from extra firm, not soft, tofu. One quarter block of tofu contains 81 g or 553 mg of calcium. Soy sauce, soy oil, and soy milk are not good sources of calcium or genistein. Other sources of vegetable protein include soy butter, peanut butter, and nuts (peanuts, almonds, walnuts, and pecans have heart-healthy benefits in addition to protein) and dried (or canned) beans and lentils mixed with brown rice. If you're ovo-vegetarian, have eggs or egg whites; whole grains such as barley, quinoa, and buckwheat; amaranth (loaded with protein); or flaxseed and unsalted seeds such as sunflower and pumpkin.

To my clients who are actors and singers concerned with slimming—as well as reducing mucus congestion to attain a bell-shaped high C—I recommend adding a scoop of protein powder (egg, whey, or other) to one-half glass of pineapple juice and water daily. Avoid orange juice (which is sweet and acidic) to reduce digestive discomfort.

Mushrooms and Fungi: Super Protein or Distant Relatives?

Edible mushrooms are a great high-protein, high-energy food. Don't try looking outside after a rain to find them—just go to www.fungi.com or www.winghopfung.com online. If you analyzed the molecular structure of mushrooms and fungi that grow on or near trees, such as Chinese "tree ears," you would find that they are more like humans than plants. Cooked mushrooms are powerful health foods. Never eat any sort of mushroom raw, because it is the cooking that releases its potent disease-killing properties. (See Chapter 4 for more information.)

Asian mushrooms are especially full of polysaccharides (concentrated sugars) that explode with energy. Diets rich in mushrooms and fungi are one reason, along with eating soy products, drinking green tea, and riding bicycles, that many Chinese and Japanese people stay slim. Mushrooms such as shiitake, maitake, ling zhi, and tree ears are high-protein foods with a big plus: according to an ever-increasing body of international research, Asian mushrooms prevent illness, including cancer and heart disease. A high-protein, low-fat diet never had it so good.

Dr. Andrew Weil, an outspoken advocate of medicinal mushrooms, always backs up his dietary suggestions with solid scientific research. At the conference, he enjoys praising some of his favorite foods, especially green tea and Asian mushrooms. He takes 60 drops of Stamets 7 Mushroom Blend daily as a high-protein energy boost. Asian mushrooms offer positive protection against environmental poisons, including radiation. Dr. Weil looks slim and more vibrant every time I see him—proof that cooked mushrooms and extracts are an excellent source of protein for health and beauty.

Live Clean and Sprout

The high carb, fruit, and veggie group tends to look starved and peaked. You may wonder if their zest for life resembles stale beansprouts. They may look squeaky clean, but can they deal with big-city stress or an active sex life? So how can we enhance our physical beauty and animal magnetism while eating a chilled-out, low-protein diet? If you have weak digestion, a raw diet can lead to fatigue, hypoglycemia, and depression. However, after recent threats of terrorism especially from pollution, germs, and poisons, you can feel most assured of clean food, it you grow it in a jar. (See how to grow sprouts on page 42.)

It takes a strong digestion to cope with raw-food diets. Sprouts are excellent live foods packed with beautifying vitamins and enzymes. However, until digestion is strengthened, sprouts can increase constipation, headaches, and gout. I add warming spices and herbs such as ginger, pepper, cardamom, mint, and dried orange peel to tea. Parsley, dandelion, and laxative herbs such as aloe vera gel in green tea also help eliminate excess acid. Oatstraw, nettle, and red clover teas are all high in nutrition and are alkalinizing. Don't neglect your supplements, including folic acid, vitamin B12, iron and a multivitamin and mineral combination. In addition, an energy-boosting herbal combination such as Chinese, American, and Siberian ginsengs can support energy and circulation. Enhancing circulation always improves sexual energy (see foot massage directions on pages 58 and 112).

Diet Options and Your Tongue

Numerous diet options are confusing. How can you know which one works best for you? A traditional Asian doctor would look at your tongue to assess your metabolism. Your tongue is a mirror of your vitality. If you are weak or tired and have a pale, scalloped tongue, indicating slow metabolism, then rich foods and animal fats can hamper digestion to make you feel stuffed. If you have a pale tongue, eating more carbohydrates can push your blood sugar balance into hypoglycemia.

If you have a dry, red tongue or chronic hunger or thirst, which indicates dehydration, inflammation, and a fast metabolism, then the best foods for you are cooling and high in antioxidants; iron; vitamins B12 and B6, found in green vegetables; dark colored fruits, such as blueberries, cherries, and strawberries; green tea; and easily digested low-fat proteins. A diet of meat and oils could lead to indigestion, circulation troubles, hypertension, and chronic pain from excess acid. Eating what's right for you turns a slimming diet into a longevity diet.

The Long-Life Slimming Diet

A long-life diet is easy to digest, nourishing, and contains minimal pollutants. More people in Japan live to be 100 years or older than anywhere on earth. They drink pots of hot green tea and eat primarily white rice, fish, seaweeds, a few fresh fruits, many vegetables, some seeds and nuts, and a cleansing fiber called konnyaku that is made into noodles. They favor tumeric root and soy products, including fermented soy tempeh, which tends to balance over- or underproduction of estrogen. Of course, hot tubs also reduce stress!

Eating wisely requires planning. My favorite diet authority is Dr. Bernard Jensen, who has written numerous excellent books on nutrition and has saved the lives of thousands. You can find sources for his products and books at the back of this book. Dr. Jensen's basic daily diet simply consists of two fruits, six vegetables, one protein (such as eggs, fish, or tofu), and one starch (such as pasta, potato, or banana). Fruit and tea make a nice cleansing breakfast. Vegetables and starch or protein work well together. Avoid eating fruit with either protein or starch because it inevitably leads to indigestion. Dr. Jensen often combines foods for their mineral content. For arthritis, he recommends dried black California mission figs and goat cheese. Delicious! It combines potassium, sodium, and calcium necessary for joint comfort. If you want to lose weight and protect your joints, add Dr. Jensen's Mt. Capra Goat Whey powder to yogurt as a meal. To make it slimming, add a salad or lightly steamed greens.

A weight-loss tea is easy to use because you can drink it all day. A good tasting slimming tea is called Get Svelte! made by Yin/Yang Sisters. It combines hawthorn and cinnamon with herbs that spark energy and clear your senses. It reduces water retention and sluggish digestion fast. Drink 1–3 cups daily. After adding the above sources of clean protein, vitamins, minerals, and digestive herbs to your diet, you will feel ready for a spot slimming routine.

Spot Slimming the Middle, Seat, and Thighs

Most of us carry extra fat and inches in the "bread basket." The following routine slims with herbs normally used to destroy parasites and poisons from the digestive tract. The herbs speed digestion, enhance absorption, and stimulate high energy. That reduces water weight and cellulite. None of the following herbs damage necessary intestinal bacteria the way using an antibiotic medicine might. However, it will be beneficial to add acidophilus or yogurt daily to enhance absorption.

I recommend following this procedure (unless you are pregnant) for at least three to six months while observing the basic high-energy diet. The payoff will surprise you—fewer allergies, reduced sugar cravings, and less depression, as well as weight loss. You will probably lose inches before pounds. The herbs help to tone abdominal muscles. If you have intestinal parasites, chronic mucus congestion in the digestive tract, or wheezing asthma, you will immediately feel better with this program. Anyone who has regularly combined meat with dairy products or fish with eggs or dairy is more likely to have parasites, whether or not they have symptoms. People with colitis or irritable bowel should use caution.

A singer, who I will call Sheila, never had parasites—only a sweet craving, monthly PMS, and water retention. After adding digestive herbs and foods to her diet for seven to ten days between each period, she prevented additional weight gain, lessened her food addictions, and lost a total of "five incredibly ugly inches that were ruining her life."

Digestive Herbs for a Slimmer Waistline

I recommend using a concentrated herbal extract such as Soothing Balance, a Long Hay Flat brand Chinese herbal extract, made and distributed by East

Earth Trade Winds in Redding, California (go to www.eastearthtrade.com). An herbal extract often works faster and stronger than taking pills or brewing a tea. You can slip the bottle into your purse or briefcase.

Soothing Balance is digestive bitters such as the after-dinner digestives enjoyed in Europe. However, it is a modification of a traditional Chinese formula called Xiao Yao Wan (Free and Easy Wanderer). Because it regulates digestion and blood sugar balance, it can be used for stomach problems, menstrual and digestive cramps, as well as for depression and irritability. A 1-ounce bottle of Soothing Balance contains buplerum, dong quai, paeoniae, atractylodis, poria, mint, licorice root, moutan, gardenia, ligustrum, gastrodia, cyperus buds, and ginger.

For our purposes, I recommend 8–10 drops added to a little water and taken with or after meals at least twice daily long term. You will notice your sweet cravings change for the better after using the digestive bitters for one week or less. It can remain your main remedy while slimming. If and when you are ready, you can continue to the next stage, which is extreme cleansing.

Extreme Cleansing: Anti-Parasite Herbs

Whether or not you have intestinal parasites or excess mucus, the antiseptic herbs used to eliminate these problems will speed slimming in your problem areas. However, parasites are easy to get—from some of the best restaurants as well as from eating street foods anywhere.

Once in Bangkok I ate in an elegant restaurant, a large traditional home with a garden. The food was delicious. The waiters were friendly. Thai love songs wafted through the air. I, in a devil-may-care mood, ordered iced coffee. The pond life trapped inside the ice cubes melted into my coffee, and I suffered later. Remember: water is never boiled to make ice. Typical symptoms of intestinal parasites may include cramps, diarrhea, constipation, jellylike or mucusy stools, and extreme lethargy. Or you may have no symptoms at all. The best way to avoid parasites is to make sure everything you eat is carefully prepared and fully cooked. Drink bottled water in questionable areas. Also, parasites can be transmitted from person to person when careful cleaning habits are not observed.

The best time to take the antiparasite herbs is at mealtimes. Before bed may be too stimulating. Aquilaria 22 and Artestatin have no unpleasant side effects. Combined, they cover a broad spectrum of parasites and protozoa, such as entamoeba histolytica, giardia, shigella, and diverticular disorders. Aquilaria 22 relieves chronic constipation. Artestatin has been used for acute attacks of vomiting and diarrhea caused by contaminated foods and water. You might take two of each tablet with meals daily. Email lethah@earthlink. net for advice.

HIV-infected or highly sensitive people can start with one Artestatin per day and increase to 2 tablets three times daily over a three-week period. Supplement these or any antiparasite herbal medicines with acidophilus. I add powdered acidophilus to yogurt before bed.

If you prefer using western herbs, Hannah Kroeger combines three remedies to make a strong antiparasite treatment. They can be warming and irritating for some but work well for people with chills, weakness, or poor liver function. For that reason, I combine them with lots of raw peeled apples. Kroeger's antiparasite regime is Wormwood combination, Rascal, and clove capsules. Wormwood combination contains black walnut leaf and male fern root, which cleanse the colon. Wormwood is often recommended for malaria as well as parasites. Rascal contains garlic, pumpkin seeds, cayenne, thyme, and cramp bark. Clove is a strong digestive stimulant that destroys parasites. All three capsules tend to have inflammatory side effects.

You will likely need to add laxative herbs such as aloe vera gel. I take ¼ or more cups daily in lots of water or green tea to help wash the parasite herbs through. If you don't add cooling laxative herbs, the Kroeger antiparasite herbs may increase nervousness, hunger, water retention, or insomnia. The herbs are too drying and heating for someone with stomach ulcers, a hyperthyroid condition, skin blemishes, or rosacea: proceed with caution.

After one month of antiparasite and colon-cleansing herbs, you may feel quite energized and your mental focus may improve. You will probably need to add aloe vera gel to water or tea in order to reduce excess acid, appetite, and insomnia. I sometimes add cooling oldenlandia diffusa capsules, a bitter herb that cleanses the liver, lungs, and urinary tract. I often add extra laxative herbs including cascara sagrada capsules.

To soothe stomach irritation, add a tea made with ¼ teaspoon each of powdered cumin, coriander, and fennel seeds. This can be added to aloe gel, yogurt, or green tea to soothe excess acid and facial flushing. I also like Balsam Pear (dried bitter melon) tea, which you can order from online sources listed at the back of the book or find in some Chinese groceries. A few people enjoy steaming raw bitter melon and sliced garlic as a side dish. Do not sweeten it even if it makes your mouth pucker. Bitter melon is anti-inflammatory and antiviral, and helps cleanse all impurities. It is recommended for diabetes. You can also add a handful of Balsam Pear Bitter Melon tea to cooking. Order it online from www.winghopfung.com.

Herbs and Massage To Ease Water
and Food Retention

If antiparasite herbs seem too complicated for you, at least increase your use of dandelion to 16–20 capsules daily. Dandelion has broad-reaching cleansing benefits. One woman I know, who routinely swallowed 16 dandelion capsules throughout the day, lost 40 pounds and a fibroid in several months. Mint is digestive, stimulating, and soothing for heartburn. Mint gel capsules are easy to find as a dried tea or in East Indian markets. The oil is sold in a small green capsule. Make sure you follow the directions on the bottle.

Drinking yarrow tea soothes the stomach. Dr. Yves Requena, an endocrinologist living in Aix en Provence, France, and author of several books on Chinese herbal medicine, once told me that yarrow and sarsaparilla (both diuretic) increase natural progesterone. He recommends them for water retention and fibroids. They are gentle and safe. Dandelion and yarrow are useful for spot reducing in the abdominal area because they are cleansing and balancing for both men and women. I would start with 4 capsules each of dandelion, yarrow, and sarsaparilla or a cup of tea made by brewing each herb.

A Tummy-Slimming Massage

This massage uses acupuncture meridians to relax the abdominal area and reduce nervous hunger and acidity. It works well for PMS sugar blues.

Sit comfortably in a chair and gently push with the palms of your hands on the front of the abdomen in order to release the diaphragm downward. Inhale into the lower abdomen, and as you exhale gently push downward from ribs, along the inner thighs to the knees. Massage around the top and behind the knees.

With your palms, apply firm pressure along the inside of each thigh for 5 minutes so that you can feel abdominal and leg tension release. Continue firmly massaging the calf down to the ankle. Massage all around the ankle top, sides, and achilles tendon. Massage your feet. You might do this relaxing yet invigorating massage while in a bath.

Japanese Slimming Fibers

Chitosan, Japanese crab shell capsules, make a slimming fiber. Konnyaku or Konjak capsules are widely used by Japanese people to lose weight and reduce cholesterol. You can't argue with the statistics: Japanese people as a whole are slim and healthy despite stress, pollution, and the stock market. Certain experts think that dietary fibers reduce fat-soluble vitamins and cause calcium excretion. If you use a cleansing fiber, it may be wise to supplement your diet with vitamins and minerals. In my experience, chitosan and konnyaku are slimming to the midsection because they absorb mucus congestion and speed digestion and elimination. They are not appetite suppressors but targeted cleansers.

A Quick Fix Program for Spot Slimming

Choose a day when you can cleanse without interruption. Have a breakfast of hot green tea, watermelon, and raw celery. The rest of the day drink Yin/Yang Sisters Get Svelte! Instant Beverage. Eat cleansing green, yellow, and orange vegetables. You might even fast on baked pumpkin or pumpkin pie filling, which is satisfying like a carbohydrate but contains fewer calories. Follow each meal with 1 capsule each of *Cascara sagrada* (laxative) and hawthorn berry (reduces cholesterol and fat), and a diuretic pill such as Chroma Slim Water Pills, which contains potassium and horsetail, parsley, paprika, uva ursi, buchu, cornsilk, juniper, and bromelain. A substitute is a cup of parsley and tarragon tea.

Be sure to support your nutrition and blood sugar with 100 mg of zinc and a combination of B vitamins with C and mixed trace minerals. A mega-dose of vitamin C strengthens adrenal energy (and the willpower to lose weight) as it cleanses the body. Use a high-quality vitamin C pill that is no larger than 500 mg. Take one pill with adequate water every hour during one day for a total of no more than 10 pills. It flushes impurities while it strengthens vitality. More than 500 mg of vitamin C taken all at once is lost in urine.

A supplement of L. carnitine reduces harmful fats that lead to heart trouble. If you exercise regularly, follow directions recommended for body builders. Otherwise, take the lowest dose. Add at least ¼ cup of aloe vera gel to juice, green tea, or water and drink it anytime you are hungry. Aloe settles the stomach and removes acidity, which is often mistaken for hunger.

Extreme Cleansing

A daily diet of vegetable juices and a cleansing enema have become a typical alternative medical treatment for cancer. A modified version of this is useful for occasional spot slimming. Barring illness or pregnancy, consider using this simple but dramatic routine during a semi-fast for extreme cleansing. It especially slims the middle and thighs. If your blood sugar is low (hypoglycemia) or if you feel weak or spacy, this program is too strong for you at this time.

Either avoid breakfast or eat one sort of fresh mucus-cleansing fruit such as pineapple, papaya, or apple and green tea. Wait for at least 2 hours then give yourself an enema made with two cups of lukewarm, pure (not tap) water and up to ¼ cup of aloe vera gel. After an enema, take a capsule of acidophilus orally to rebalance the colon's digestive energy. Increase the dose if you develop constipation. The aloe vera enema cleanses acidic impurities from the colon and blood to prevent blemishes. Wait at least two hours before resuming eating, then drink only vegetable juice. If blemishes develop because impurities have been released into the blood, add a dose or two of a skin-cleansing herbal pill such as the Chinese patent remedy Lien Chiao Pai Tu Pien or Skin Balance, made by Health Concerns. Use such remedies between meals as needed.

If for any reason you give yourself a daily enema or colon irrigation, you can easily add Schuessler's 12 homeopathic tissue salts (which are essential minerals) to the water in order to prevent illness and aging. If you plan to cleanse on a long-term basis, drink a tonic tea such as Yin/Yang Sisters Gorgeous You Instant Beverage.

Cellulite

In my weekly internet health column at www.winghopfung.com I began an informal study on cellulite, drawing data from mostly women participants who ranged between the ages of 20 to 70 years. The women ordered what they needed for the study directly from the website, which is maintained by the largest store selling Chinese ginseng and other products in Los Angeles.

The top-selling anticellulite herb soon became laminaria seaweed. Laminaria, high in potassium and iodine, stimulates cleansing, reduces water retention, and tones thyroid action. It reduces mucus congestion and poor metabolism, which underlie cellulite. An easy way to use it is in pills called Laminaria 4, made by Health Concerns.

Results covering over 80 women came in during the first six months after the observation began. All responses were enthusiastic. Nearly all participants lost from 1 to 3 inches from the waist and anywhere from 10 to 60 pounds. The participants lowered dietary fats and added the following herbs daily: 6–9 pills of Laminaria 4; 6 cups of green tea; 3 cups of Get Svelte! Yin/Yang Sisters Instant Beverage; and 40 drops daily of ginkgo extract. After seven weeks, most participants reported substantial weight loss, improved muscle tone, increased energy, as well as better mental clarity and overall work performance.

Especially for Men

Men tend to hold fat in the abdominal area. Women generally become pear-shaped, with their weight in the hips. In addition to following my suggestions, including daily doses of Soothing Balance extract, homeopathic pulsatilla 30C is recommended for mucus congestion and food addictions. The remedy feels like a soothing stomach massage. It improves breathing and energy. If you feel suffocated in a stuffy room, if you want to break out and smell the roses but you can't smell anything from sinus congestion, homeopathic pulsatilla 30C can help "clear the air." One dose is five pills taken as needed between meals. For chronic problems, use at least five doses daily. Some people prefer taking it along with Soothing Balance extract. You might follow the One-Day Program several days a week each month.

Lola's Way

Did you ever think about the quantity of memories stored in fat? Losing weight gives you a chance to become younger and wiser. Lola Montez quipped, "Many a rich lady would give all her fortune to possess the expanded chest and rounded arm of her kitchen girl. Well, she might have had both, by the same amount of exercise and spare living."

Try the following exercise: think back to a time when you were an ideal weight or very healthy. What were your interests and ambitions then? How have they changed? What have you gained from age, wealth, and experience? Spare living is not poverty. Pay close attention to how you eat and with whom. Create pleasant dining experiences with candles, flowers, and a sparkling digestive liquor you make at home. Steep about 20 pills or up to ½ cup of your favorite spot-slimming raw herbs from this chapter in 1 liter of gin. Be sure to add as ingredients digestive bitters such as dandelion root and pungent dried orange peel. Keep it airtight for two weeks before decanting. After meals, add 10 drops of the slimming elixir to seltzer.

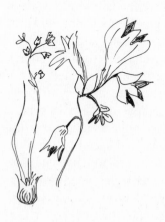

7

Your Body Beautiful

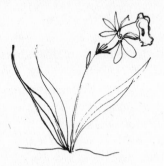

*"'As the twig is bent, the tree's inclined,' is quite as true of
the body as of the mind."*
—LOLA MONTEZ

Your shape is an energy issue. Fat is weak. Fit is sleek. We can't reduce our total number of fat cells, we can only reduce water retention, which slims their size. Most women want gazelle-like, long, and firm muscles, while men work for round and full biceps, a washboard stomach, and rock-solid thighs. Long or round, muscles require nutrients to insure strength and smooth action. Chinese herbs recommended to enhance athletic performance keep you in shape, whether or not you compete, because they support endurance and vitality. We have covered several adaptogens that reduce stress and illness in Chapter 3. To use them for endurance requires a higher or more concentrated dosage in order to facilitate exercise and speed recovery time. Careful selection and attention paid to side effects is important when using a higher dose. This chapter can be your guide to recharging your muscles naturally.

Ask a weight trainer to describe muscle strength and the answer will probably be the number of pounds you can press at the gym. My brother, Dr. Eric Hadady, former light-heavyweight Mr. New Mexico and now a chiropractor in Albuquerque, has described strength as "having consistent stamina more than power; the ability to make progressive gains at the gym." He (gorgeous)

works out at the gym as often as his busy schedule permits and uses adaptogenic herbs, including Chinese and raw tienchi ginsengs for energy and
muscle tone and ling zhi mushroom extract for joint comfort and endurance.
I have talked to women boxers, runners, tennis pros, golfers, and hikers who
agree with Eric: stamina (without muscle aches or tremors) is what counts for
performance on the playing court as well as on the dance floor.

Muscles require nourishment and support from herbs because they support
posture, balance, and internal organs. The stage manager for New York City's
Rockettes once told me that the whole idea of "showgirls" has totally changed
in the last 50 years. "The girls are athletic," he said. "Precision dancing is an
expression of their athleticism." Several of the women are professional massage therapists who use energy-enhancing herbs from this chapter on a daily
basis. You too can be a Rockette: the Avon products website (avon.com) sells
the Rockettes' kick yourself into shape exercise video. It's a scream.

Secrets of the Olympians

In 2004, countless numbers of us will become "Olympics addicts," watching
beautiful bodies in competition. Chinese herbs that build vitality offer exceptionally good results for anyone who wants an athletic body. Energy-boosting
herbs help prevent injury and fatigue. That goes for demanding professions
of all sorts. The Chinese women's soccer team excels during the world cham-
pionship games, considering that the players are generally much smaller than
those on other teams. Chinese operas last for as long as nine hours with little
interruption. That calls for stamina!

In your local health-food store and around the world on the internet, you
will find Chinese herbal combinations, often including various ginsengs,
astragalus, and other adaptogenic tonics. A number of highly successful
American manufacturers of herbal supplements have been founded by American acupuncturists. McZand and East Earth Trade Winds products are backed
by American research done at clinics associated with their companies. Once,
for a magazine article I was writing, I e-mailed Michael Czehatowski, founder
of East Earth Trade Winds with a question. He answered from China, where
he was doing advanced studies in acupuncture. Among energy-enhancing
products, he recommends Dragon 'seng, a combination of ginseng and powerful tonic herbs designed to be used daily.

According to Jerry Wu, founder of Drako, a California and China–based
manufacturer of full-spectrum standardized water-processed herbs, many
Chinese Olympic athletes he has worked with use Chinese, American, and
Siberian ginsengs, cordyceps, and herbs that increase circulation, including
tienchi (a.k.a. pseudoginseng powder). For a testosterone boost, they simmer

epimedium leaf with lycium fruit as a tea. Adding a few of these herbs daily can power up life and limb.

Chinese tonic herbs, which enhance the functioning of internal organs, do not offer exactly the same results for everyone. People vary. A lot also depends on how herbs are combined and used. If adding energy and endurance herbs makes you feel temporarily off center or spacy, your digestion may be weak. Especially in the beginning, I recommend using a digestive remedy with meals. One good remedy is Vitality Combination, which contains poria, ginger, atractylodes, and paeonia and is made by Sanjiu 999 company, one of China's largest herb manufacturers. It is distributed by East Earth Trade Winds. Poria and atractylodes slenderize and ginger builds energy.

Chinese energy-boosting herbs improve performance, endurance, grace, and freedom from pain partly because they enable you to deal with stress. Some of the most popular tonics combine several forms of ginseng, astragalus, epimedium, and lycium fruit. Although they can be used separately as pills, teas or cooked in soup, their best results are in herbal combinations. For example, Chinese (ren shen), American (si yang seng), and Siberian (ciwijia) ginsengs can be combined to strengthen muscles, increase circulation, and improve glucose management. For maximum performance, other adaptogenic herbs such as *Schizandra chinensis* (wu wei zi) or *Astragalus membranaceous* (huang qi) can be added to reduce energy loss from strain and excess sweating.

Combining energizing herbs along with herbs that hold in vitality is a bit like putting a lid on a jar of explosives. The resulting dynamo fuels internal organs to ensure strength and coordination. Herbal combinations such as these enhance endurance and cut recovery time because they are balanced. Some herbs are stimulating; others replenish fluids.

Power Up Your Workouts

As we learned in Chapter 3, adaptogens enable us to overcome extreme climate, pollution, fatigue, or nervous tension. If you use adaptogens such as ginseng to energize your workouts on a regular basis, take a dose during mid-morning and mid-afternoon as well as half an hour before your workout. Avoid all tonic herbs, especially ginseng, if you catch a cold or flu.

Chinese ginseng (a.k.a. red ginseng, *Panax ginseng,* and in Chinese ren shen), the best-known adaptogen, is considered warming: it stimulates metabolism, energy, and resistance to cold weather. It reverses chronic fatigue, weakness, low blood pressure, weak sexuality, and poor memory. Use it only if you have a pale tongue and chronic chills. Avoid it if you have a dry, red tongue, thirst, nervousness, headache, or fever. To warm the body and build resistance, you might eat 1 tablespoon of cooked root with meals once daily or drink the tea anytime to speed digestion of proteins and carbs. Many ginseng pills, extracts, and combinations are available.

Your dosage of Chinese ginseng depends on your level of fatigue, your blood pressure, your size, and, for women, menopausal factors. Start with the smallest recommended dosage and watch for these signs of overdose—thirst, dizziness or headache, insomnia, crankiness, and reduced body fluids (dark urine, reduced semen, or vaginal dryness). You can balance the heating and drying effects of Chinese ginseng by combining it with cooling, moistening American ginseng.

American or white ginseng (a.k.a *Panax quinquefolium,* and in Chinese si yang seng) reverses dryness. It replenishes saliva and reduces thirst. American ginseng acts as a stimulant for people burned out from stress, sugar and salt addictions, excess sweating, or chronic fever conditions. Singers have told me that American ginseng tea helps them to sing long performances without throat irritations. Several of my clients, who as college students practically lived on coffee and donuts, have said that American ginseng reduced their sugar cravings. If you have a dry, red tongue, drink American ginseng tea all day, especially at the gym. To refresh your breath, melt some instant American ginseng tea in your mouth.

Neutral ginseng or codonopsis (in Chinese dang shen) is neither warming nor cooling, but speeds metabolism and turns fat into muscle. Andrew Gaeddert, founder of Health Concerns and author of several books, including *Healing Digestive Disorders*, recommends for muscle weakness codonopsis along with Chinese ginseng and astragalus, an energy and immune-boosting herb. When I called Andrew at his Get Well Clinic in Oakland, California, where he works with 89-year-old herbalist Dr. Fung Fung, he reported that he had recently treated some 15 athletes, including several triathletes and a world record-holding runner. Their chronic fatigue and endurance problems improved dramatically within two to four weeks with a combination of astragalus, Siberian ginseng (*Eleuthero ginseng*), *Ganoderma lucidum,* and codonopsis. The dosage was 3 pills three times daily.

Acupuncturists including Dr. Janet Zand, author and founder of McZand Herbal Inc., recommend ganoderma (ling zhi) for recovery after painful workouts. Zand has treated many athletes including medal-winning American and Canadian Olympic runners and swimmers. Her clients reported that after a tough workout they felt physically spent. Within one week after using a combination of 350 mg of highly concentrated (10:1) ganoderma extract combined with a smaller amount of cordyceps and 100 mg Siberian ginseng each four times daily, the athletes had no problems with recovery and could do two consecutive workouts.

Ganoderma is best suited for cardiovascular enrichment. When you buy the dry mushroom from Chinese herbs shops, have the herbalists chop it into pieces or make a powder. Simmer a handful in a crockpot of water for six hours or take 6–10 capsules daily between meals.

Testosterone in a Leaf

Epimedium sagittatum (yin yang huo), an herbal precursor to testosterone, treats sore lower back, weak legs, sexual impotence, and reduced resistance to cold weather. Epimedium has heating effects so that it should be combined with cooling moistening herbs such as lycium fruit (gou qi zi) or fo-ti (*Polygonum multiflorum,* in Chinese he shou wu). Take a handful of each and simmer them in one quart of water for 20 minutes. Drink the tea between meals. Do not eat garlic or hot spices that day and be wary of overdose discomforts—flushed feeling, dizziness, or insomnia. It will not make you feel sexually antsy, just stronger. Men and women can use epimedium as a tea without any side effects as long as they do not have fever, headaches, sparse burning urine, or other inflammatory conditions.

Beware of Yohimbe, an herbal aphrodisiac that increases testosterone. It is too inflammatory for gym use. Known as an aphrodisiac, the herb can give you a headache or an erection when you don't need it. To avoid gym freak-outs, yohimbe must never be mixed with alcohol or any sort of drug, especially psychological or psychiatric drugs, because it exaggerates mental and emotional imbalances.

Performance-Packed Chinese Herbs

Individual dosage of Chinese herbs varies according to individual needs. For a tea (leaves or berries) steep for five minutes. When simmering for at least 30 minutes to make a decoction (roots, leaves, mushrooms, or berries), use no more than one root (or 200 mg) of each herb.

Herb	Symptoms to Treat	Area of Benefit	Result of Overdose
Chinese ginseng	Pale tongue, listless, chills	Energy, endurance	Headache, insomnia
American ginseng	Thirst	Endurance	Nausea
Neutral ginseng (codonopsis)	Flab	Metabolism	—
Siberian ginseng	Exhaustion	Nerves	Insomnia
Raw Tienchi ginseng	Bruises	Circulation	Chills
Cordyceps	Asthma, weakness	Energy	—

continued

Herb	Symptoms to Treat	Area of Benefit	Result of Overdose
Ganoderma	Slow recovery	Immunity	—
Astragalus	Excess sweating	Immunity	—
Epimedium tea	Backache	Vitality	Headache
Lycium fruit tea	Bloodshot eyes	Liver	Diarrhea
Polygonum multifl.	Gray hair	Liver and blood	Diarrhea
Schizandra	Excess sweating	Energy	—

Athletic Competition

Meals for a serious athlete can be a different experience than for most of us. A body-builder diet is aimed to increase strength, endurance, and muscle mass and to reduce water weight. In general, protein supports muscle synthesis and carbohydrates fuel workouts. Each come with certain problems. Proteins require good digestion and elimination of acids. Carbohydrates increase water retention. If you want to reduce water weight, reduce sodium (table salt) and "wet" carbohydrates such as pasta and increase astringent (water-absorbing) carbohydrates such as oats.

Increased protein reduces water weight and increases muscle mass. One gram of carbohydrates holds 9 calories as opposed to 1 gram of protein, which holds 4. For the average man, 1 gram of protein daily is required per kilo (2.26 pounds) of body weight. However, for athletic training, more protein is required—up to 1 gram of low-fat protein per pound from chicken, lean beef, whey, soy, or beans and rice.

Men and women might use the same nutritional supplements except the dosage should vary. For example, more than 1000 mg of Siberian ginseng daily may increase testosterone in women, possibly leading to unwanted facial hair, menstrual troubles, or fibroids. Men, unless they develop headaches or inflammation, can use from 2000 to 5000 mg daily to harden muscles and increase strength and endurance. I would add cleansing and digestive aids to improve absorption as well as large daily doses of papaya and pineapple enzymes for pain reduction. Those enzymes eliminate toxic material and inflammation from the joints and muscles while they increase healing of injuries.

A Beautiful Body is Pain Free

Even if your daily workout is in front of a computer screen, the following remedies will help prevent carpal tunnel syndrome as well as other circulation-related pain and fatigue. Throughout the day between meals, sip bottled water and one of these homeopathic remedies:

- *Arnica montana* 30C for bruising or stress-injury pain
- *Ruta graveolens* 30C for tendonitis
- *Aesculus hippocastanum* 30C (homeopathic horse chestnut) for varicose veins and hemorrhoids

Horse chestnut (the herb) helps shrink swollen blood vessels, but is not recommended for high blood pressure. The homeopathic form is safer to use because the dose is minute. It readily penetrates to the blood and is excreted when it's not necessary. Homeopathic calc. fluor. 30C (calcium fluoride) is also recommended for varicose veins. You can also use it if you have bleeding gums or loose teeth. It is safe for weak, elderly people as well as for anyone whose nutritional habits prevent calcium absorption. Homeopathic arnica also comes in a convenient ointment you can apply directly to sore muscles and bruises. A fine brand called Traumeel is made in Germany by Biologische and distributed in Albuquerque, New Mexico, by Heel/BHI Inc.

Jason Natural Cosmetic Company in Culver City, California, makes many wholesome products for health and beauty. Not far from Hollywood, their company was originally started to service the beauty needs of stars. Today they have more than 40 years of experience and make a large line of products using nutritional raw herbal and plant materials, aromatherapy, organic botanicals, and food-grade nutraceuticals from around the world. Jason's Cap-Max6 cream naturally combines capsaicin, echinacea, and arnica to create a highly active, deep penetrating pain reliever. This product provides a quick delivery to relieve joint stiffness, muscle soreness, or sprains.

Jason's Tea Tree Oil Therapeutic Mineral Gel is a deep penetrating, cooling therapeutic gel that helps relax tight and aching muscles, bringing relief. Its vegetarian formula contains no animal fats, mineral oil, petrolatum, or paraffin wax. It is greaseless, stainless, and pleasant to use. This is Jason's "deep cold therapy" for the treatment of pain and injuries.

A Quick Fix for Performance Excellence

A daily pill supplement made up of Chinese ginseng and royal jelly is a fast, convenient way to maintain energy and endurance for most people. Chinese ginseng is balanced enough to take for prevention of weakness unless inflammatory pain or fevers are present. Royal jelly is an excellent, beautifying source of B vitamins. Available in Chinese supermarkets, herb shops, and online, the pills or liquid extract can be taken with or between meals for added nutrition.

Normally, the recommended dose is 3 pills daily. If you find ginseng and royal jelly to be too stimulating, take 1 capsule daily after breakfast. Avoid it at night. During the day until 8:00 P.M., eat five or six light meals in order to speed your metabolism. If you fast or eat infrequently during the day, your body's natural reaction will be to slow its metabolism. Drink liquids between meals so that they will not weaken digestion.

Steroid Substitutes

Athletes have asked me about natural substitutes for steroid drugs to increase workout strength and time. People with arthritic pain and joint deformity also want a substitute for damaging pain drugs. Steroid drugs have been known to strip bone density and have long-term weakening effects for adrenal vitality, which can impact on immunity, sexuality, and mood.

The most popular synthesized supplement now is creatine monohydrate. Any protein naturally contains creatine. It enters the cells and is converted into muscle fuel. It tricks the body into storing more fuel than it normally would. It is transformed into ATP, a molecule that has three phosphate high-energy bonds. As ATP is broken down, energy is released into muscles. It is like a fuel in disguise. By taking creatine, you fool the body into taking in more muscle fuel than normal. In that way, a 5-gram dose of creatine is like eating a steak.

A problem associated with using creatine is that it gives off the same nitrate wastes as any protein. While increasing muscle fuel with it, you have to consume extra water to wash away the wastes accumulated from protein synthesis. Most body builders, informally trained in nutrition, are advised to load up with creatine (20 grams per day per week then cut back). But a safer way to consume it is to use 4–5 grams of the powder per day for one month. It lasts longer and is easier on the body.

The side effects can be water retention and headache. For that reason, women, who tend to retain water or suffer from PMS, will benefit less from creatine. My body builder brother Eric believes that creatine, without increasing endurance, can make a man feel stronger so that he can lift heavier weights and build bigger muscles. However, women need to increase their metabolism with cardiovascular workouts and isolated muscle resistance exercises to *tone* muscles instead of working out with heavy weights. Heavy weight-training using many pounds of resistance and the synthesis of protein (from creatine) naturally causes bloating from water retention.

A number of Chinese anti-inflammatory herbs work like steroids to reduce swelling and pain without harmful side effects. One recommended for its tonic properties is sea cucumber. The easiest way to take it is as Sea-Q pills made by Health Concerns, which requires a recommendation from an herbalist. It acts as a moistening tonic that is useful, in combination with other herbs, for arthritis and sexual impotence. The side effects can include bloating and diarrhea for people with weak digestion.

Especially for Men

Natural testosterone herbs such as cuscuta and epimedium increase the body's ability to withstand fatigue and backache. They support healthy adrenal function. However, they are more than energy tonics. Because they increase natural testosterone, they also increase male sexual traits—beards, low voice, aggression, increased sex drive, and hard muscles. If used to excess, they can cause dizziness, headache, fever, skin blemishes, muscle spasms, irritability, and a general overheated reaction. Strength and courage don't come from increased heat and drive, but from physical resilience and mental focus. Most often, Chinese testosterone-increasing herbs such as epimedium are combined with cooling, moistening, blood-enhancing herbs such as lycium fruit or he shou wu in order to protect internal organs and maintain balance.

Lola's Way

"There have been many instances of sedentary men, of shrunk and sickly forms, with deficient muscle and scraggly arms, who by a change of business to a vigorous outdoor exercise acquired fine robust forms." So wrote Lola Montez in *The Arts of Beauty.* It is time to take up a new sport—not your usual workout or rowing machine. Make it something sexy, expensive, and classy, such as horseback riding or playing squash at an exclusive club. One trained athlete told me that playing squash expends the most calories. Show off the great body you are developing as a result of reading this book. Appreciative glances are always inspiring.

Buy a smashing gym outfit or swimsuit. If you have a problem spending money—not an issue for Hungarian countesses—then hold a dollar bill and visualize the expensive outfit you want to buy. The dollar is symbolic. Repeat these words as a credo: "It's *only* money." Throw it out the window.

What if building the perfect body leads to unpleasant odors and stained clothing? Find help in the following chapter. Fragrance plays a key role in your personal signature.

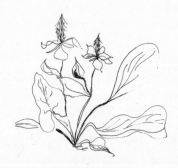

8

Fragrance from the Inside Out

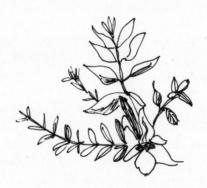

"Nothing can cure the soul but the senses, just as nothing
can cure the senses but the soul."
—Oscar Wilde

Perfume oils and ointments were prized by the early Egyptians as beauty
potions, medicines, mystical offerings to deities, and rich enticements for
lovers. Kyphi, a popular incense and medicine, combined grapes, honey,
wine, tree resins such as myrrh, and a few traditional herbs including, lemon
grass, mint, sweet flag, and cinnamon. The bitter/sweet paste was burned in
temples to chase evil spirits and drunk with wine in order to cure liver and
lung ailments. It was one of the earliest examples of fragrance being used to
enliven the senses and enhance vitality.

The Greek botanist Theophrastus (c. 372–287 B.C.), in his essay "On
Odours," listed 20 plants used for perfumes, including flowers, leaves, wood
resins, and seeds. They included lemongrass, cardamom, cinnamon, juniper
berry, dill, cyprus, iris, lily, marjoram, mint, pine, sweet flag, saffron, and
lotus.

Essential oils, currently used for aromatherapy, are pure enough for internal use as teas or inhalers. You might add them to a vaporizer, bath, lotion, or
massage and hair oils. To feel its effects, dab a drop on the top of your head

or chest. Or add 10–20 drops of a pure essential oil to water and then wash your wood floors or furniture with it to diffuse the aroma. You might vary the fragrance according to your mood, activities, or the weather. This chapter will restore the magical power of fragrance in personal alchemy: you will learn to use fragrance according to your goals. The first step is to overcome problem odors.

The Odor of Fight and Flight

Our body's natural fragrance is a byproduct of energy being converted in the cells. It involves the play of blood, fluids, and oxygen during breathing, digestion, and elimination. Emotions affect body odors because they influence cleansing and inflammation. Anger and fear are unmistakably foul smelling. A vital warning signal in the animal world, scent can mean the difference between life and death.

In China, I once stood 10 feet away from a large tiger trapped in a humiliating zoo cage. His confinement troubled us both. I chanted a Buddhist prayer to see if the tiger would be quieted. We gazed at each other during one long moment. I stood very still as he sharpened his focus. The involuntary pounding of my heart, a rise in blood pressure, fast breathing, and sweating signaled alarm. Suddenly, we recognized each other as predator and prey. I stared into his black-gold eyes as he sprang full against the cage. My nervous response was seeping through my skin as the unmistakable scent of fear.

Primitive brain reactions trigger hormones that spark fight or flight. That natural reaction is counterproductive on a date or at a job interview. To avoid unpleasant personal odors, we need to reduce impurities and the inflammatory effects of anxiety and physical stress. Here are some general suggestions.

Bad Breath

To eliminate halitosis, we need to reduce acids or inflammation produced in the stomach, lungs, nervous system, and skin. Smokers' breath has the odor of burnt flesh, which we smell as the smoker exhales. The acidic breath of fasting (or nervous stomach) comes from the release of ketones when digestive acids begin to burn. Several homeopathic remedies are helpful. Natrum sulphate 6x reduces bilious symptoms such as burping and nausea. Use it especially if you look jaundiced or are constipated. Natrum phosphate 6x reduces excess acid indigestion.

Green leafy vegetables such as kale, asparagus, and watercress enhance complexion brightness and facilitate the absorption of necessary oxygen and minerals. Cabbage in salad or raw juice is alkaline to soothe an irritated stomach. Green fresh herbs such as mint, dill, cilantro, tarragon, and parsley in salad or tea are cleansing and soothing. Cooked oatmeal is another excellent moisturizing food full of nutrients to refresh the skin, soothe aching joints, and help eliminate impurities.

Honeysuckle flowers with mint or parsley make a tea that is cleansing for the breath and relaxing. Instead of honey, use an herbal sweetener such as Chinese Lo Han Kuo instant beverage to reduce lung inflammation. You can add a cube as a sugar substitute to a coffee substitute or any tea. Other favorites are Sheshecao Beverage, crystals made with skullcap, *Oldenlandia diffusa,* and powdered pearl. That sweetener clears your complexion as it refreshes your breath. You can order them online from www.winghopfung.com.

The Burnt Smell of Caffeine

If you work under pressure and use caffeine as a stimulant, you will recognize its burnt, bitter smell as it heats your metabolism and nervous system response. Caffeine can stress circulation and respiration. One way to rid unpleasant stress odors is with a homeopathic remedy for caffeine withdrawal, insomnia, or nervous anxiety. For example, homeopathic coffea cruda 30C is a form of homeopathic coffee recommended for insomnia and anxiety.

Another antihype remedy is Caffeine Withdrawal made by Natra-Bio. Its ingredients include homeopathic chamomile, nux vomica, spanish fly, and guarana. It takes the edge off after you don't need it. Take these between meals so you can come off the ceiling and stop smelling like burned wires. Remember, if you overuse caffeine today, you may have to pay tomorrow with backache, chronic fatigue, and tooth and gum trouble.

Garlic, Onions, Odors, and Pain

Have you ended an evening or a friendship abruptly after eating raw garlic? It might be the only perennial vegetable (a member of the lily family) that can come between friends. The reason why raw garlic stays with you so long is that its odor comes through the skin as well as from the breath. Its high iodine and sulphur content can start an acidic chain reaction that can give you heartburn for days.

Garlic contains a powerful bactericide called crotonaldehyde. It kills germs, intestinal worms, and yeast—and it can just about kill your friends when you breathe on them! Steam and mash garlic and then add olive oil for cooking or salads. Or use pills that have added parsley to neutralize the odor. If you eat raw garlic and burp for hours, try calming the digestive acid by drinking up to ¼ cup liquid chlorophyll and water, ½ cup aloe vera in apple juice, or lots of laxative hot green tea.

Gas Indigestion Odors

If every food upsets your digestion (including not eating), the problem is likely a poor combination of food or candida yeast in the digestive tract. Fruits and sweets slow digestion and cause gas bubbles. Eat fruit separately from starch and proteins.

Yeast often develops after using antibiotics or birth control pills or as a result of exhaustion from drugs, surgery, or other causes. Antibiotics kill most digestive bacteria. The yeast, which is always present, takes over and eliminates necessary bacteria to make your digestion, absorption, energy, and mood suffer. Popular herbal antiyeast remedies include one drop of Australian Tea Tree oil added to water as tea and Phellostatin herbal pills, made by Health Concerns. (See herbal suggestions in my book *Personal Renewal* for eliminating candida yeast.)

Sometimes gas is aggravated by weak digestion. Chinese patent remedies such as Xiao Yao Wan or Er Chen Wan pills (up to 12 daily) or Vitality Tabs, distributed by www.eastearthtrade.com, will help. Adding ginger, mint, cardamom, and dried citrus peel to tea is also digestive. Health-food store digestive enzyme pills are useful with meals. A remedy to keep in your purse is carbo veg 30C (homeopathic charcoal), which absorbs gas. Take up to 5 doses daily as needed between meals.

Fragrance According to the Five Elements

Ancient Chinese doctors described specific body odors associated with the Five Elements—Fire, Earth, Metal, Water, and Wood—because personal fragrance helps to identify health issues and emotions. Acupuncture often releases odors associated to the Five Elements as the body detoxifies during a cooling treatment. The Chinese Five Element theory is a window to our energetic world. Its influence is compelling although most people cannot read its signs.

Most odors suggest inflammatory conditions affecting the blood or internal organs. Sickness smells bad. Acids, impurities, addictions, and poisons seep through the skin. In the following section, I describe energy and fragrance remedies for the Chinese Five Elements. The suggestions do more than mask symptoms. In each case, healing aromas can be used as incense, essential oils for internal and external use, or teas.

Compare the fragrance information in this chapter with the dietary advice in Chapter 4, Your Seasons of Beauty, and you will recognize a connection between the Five Elements and the seasons. Fire is summer or hot weather; Earth is Indian summer or humid weather; Metal is autumn or cool, dry weather; Water is winter or cold weather; and Wood is spring or allergy sea-son. Now you can use fragrances as well as foods to balance your energy and promote beauty.

Cool Fire

The Fire Element, comprised of the heart and circulatory system, has a charac-teristic burnt smell when overheated. You can get a whiff of it from people who suffer from high blood pressure, fever, hot flashes, or who are "burned-out" from stimulating addictions such as smoking. Do these statements reflect you?

- I often feel anxious.
- I have poor circulation, high cholesterol, or chest pains.
- My palms or tongue look pink or purplish.
- I chatter and giggle when nervous.
- I find it difficult to calm myself before a meeting or performance.

If you agree with three or more items, you may need to cool your Fire with any of the following: bitter salad greens, cucumber cooling drinks, up to ½ cup of aloe vera gel, green tea, evening primrose oil, or raw tienchi ginseng. A cleansing diet will help to reduce inflammation. Use homeopathic silicea 30C when under stress. It is a useful remedy for unpleasant body odors, espe-cially foot odors, resulting from a buildup of impurities, malabsorption, and stress. It removes wastes from the blood and cells, while it enhances growth of bones, strong hair, and fingernails.

Jason Natural Cosmetic makes Soothing Sports Body Wash, which is very refreshing while it cleanses chlorine, salt, and sweaty odors from the body. Specially formulated herbal ingredients such as chamomile, aloe vera, and comfrey moisturize and soothe.

Cooling, pungent fragrances counteract excess Fire. They include essen-tial oil of camphor, lavender, lemongrass, oregano, rosewood, sandalwood, spearmint, tea tree oil, and wintergreen.

Balance and Center Earth

The Earth Element, comprised of the stomach, spleen, pancreas, and flesh, has a sickly-sweet, dank smell when troubled. All odors including urine and sweat are sticky and sweet, which is characteristic of people with diabetes or excess fat.

- I crave sweets when nervous, tired, or bored.
- I wilt in humid weather.
- I get stomach troubles or diarrhea when upset.

- I feel scattered or spacy much of the time.
- I am too thin or too heavy.

If you agree with three or more items, it would be wise to protect your emotions and blood sugar balance with a sensible diet. Avoid alcohol and add oats, asparagus, yams, and beans. If you have diabetes, avoid all sweets— fruit, carrots, and beets.

Spicy or astringent fragrances are balancing for Earth. They include essential oil of anise, basil, bergamot, cinnamon, citronella, fennel, ginger, lemon, lime, orange, tangerine, ylang ylang, and vetivert.

Moisturize and Protect Metal

The Metal Element, comprised of the lungs, large intestine, and skin, requires regular moisturizing and cleansing. If inflammation builds up from stress, spicy foods and alcohol, or smoking, a putrid or metallic odor from mouth, nose, and skin will signal stress and anxiety.

- I am often thirsty or have a dry cough.
- I have dry skin or scalp, dandruff, or eczema.
- The bad taste in my mouth is like a copper penny.
- I feel short of breath or wheeze.
- I have chronic skin blemishes.

If you are overheated from diet or lifestyle, add cooling, moistening laxative greens such as green tea, bitter melon, or white rice. Simmer a handful of Chinese dried lily bulbs or ophiopogon buds cooked along with rice to ease dryness and anxiety from lung inflammation. Ching Fei Yi Huo Pien reduces cough, congestion, and dryness. You can take 4 pills twice daily between meals. American ginseng tea is refreshing.

Sweet soothing essential oils such as chamomile or vanilla are calming. Eucalyptus will feel refreshing and can help you to breathe deeper. Other useful fragrances include red thyme, peppermint, patchouli, myrrh, geranium, and juniper berry, which help clear lungs and stimulate energy.

Soften Water

The Water Element, comprised of the kidney, urinary bladder, hormones, and sexual fluids, can become overheated or stressed from exhaustion, stimulants, jet lag, and emotional upset. Inflammation gives off a spoiled fishy smell. Overstimulated adrenal energy (inflammation) can lead to excess sexual excitement, muscle tension, hyper energy, or paranoia. Whereas poor adrenal energy leads to fatigue, chronic aches, dietary binging, sexual weakness, and menstrual irregularity.

- I am always right.
- I work until I drop, then get up for more.
- I have been depressed forever.
- I am overweight and never seem to lose pounds.
- I am frequently up all night and feel sleepy during the day.

If you have worn-out adrenal energy from excess work, childbirth, or illness, you need to rebuild vitality to maintain metabolism and mental clarity. You may feel out of focus or unable to stay on track at work. Switch from coffee to tea. To sleep and reduce nerve pains, nervousness, insomnia, and excess hunger use homeopathic coffea cruda 30C (homeopathic coffee) daily.

Chinese Shou Wu Pien pills and ayurvedic Shilajit capsules are moisturizing to recondition the liver and kidneys. Both increase sexual fluids to revitalize sexuality and fertility. Such nutritive tonics slow digestion and increase mucus congestion. Avoid taking them during colds and flu.

Heavy, oily fragrances like jasmine and gardenia can relax you. If you can't sleep, valerian, a nerve sedative, may quiet excess energy. If you like its grounding, earthy fragrance, add a few drops of valerian extract to massage oil, to your bath, or on your chest.

Useful essential oils include warming stimulants such as sage, clove, geranium, and ginger or soothing herbs marjoram and lemongrass, depending on your energy and mood.

Cleanse and Nourish Wood

The Wood Element, comprised of the liver and gall bladder, affects muscles, tendons, vision, and temper. Abusing it with stimulants, drug and alcohol addictions, and anger, will overstimulate the liver to give the body a rotten smell. Notice the sudden rise in body odor during an argument.

- I fall asleep very late at night, sometimes not until 3 A.M.
- I crave rich foods, red meat, hot spices, and alcohol.
- With fatigue, my nerves and muscles ache.
- I have allergies, headaches, or arthritis.
- My vision is poor.

If you have had hepatitis, mononucleosis, or jaundice, you need to rest and rebuild your liver with lots of green vegetables and liquid chlorophyll, omega 3 and 6 fish oils, and natural vitamin A sources. A Chinese herbal supplement such as Ligan Pian pills (5 pills twice daily for up to two weeks) can be helpful to clear bile congestion and pain on the right side of the ribs. Other useful liver cleansing herbs are burdock and dandelion. They are bitter in flavor and astringent (they gather impurities to the liver so that they can be eliminated).

Another great herb for problems associated with liver damage from drugs, chemicals, and diet as well as blood and bone marrow deficiency from chemotherapy and hair loss is *Eclipta alba* (han lien cao). Health Concerns makes a serious liver-rebuilding pill called Ecliptex, which contains concentrated eclipta, milk thistle, curcuma (a form of turmeric), salvia, lycium fruit, ligustrum, bupleurum, schizandra, tienchi ginseng, tang kuei, plantago seed, and licorice root. It is recommended for rehabilitating a liver that has been weakened by environmental chemicals, pharmaceutical drugs, bad habits, and inflammatory illness such as hepatitis. If you have been exposed to toxic chemicals or are highly sensitive, start with 1 pill two or three times daily and increase to 1–3 pills three times daily for a period of at least two months.

Woodsy fragrances such as essential oil of cedar, pine, fir, or spruce are invigorating. They are particularly cheery fragrances to harmonize your home in blustery weather. Around Christmas, my apartment smells like a forest because I add essential spruce oil to water as a floor wash.

For inflammatory arthritis or a scorched-garbage body odor, add a few drops of essential oil of cooling mint or sandalwood to sunflower or walnut oil normally used for cooking. Apply it topically for body massage, to a dry flaky scalp, or on painful, swollen joints.

Prevent Excess Sweating

Spontaneous sweating such as after eating or at night can result from weakness. TCM doctors see it as a sign of imbalance. The herbs you should choose depend on the accompanying symptoms. If a person with spontaneous sweating has a red, dry tongue and excess thirst, I might recommend a moistening, blood-enhancing formula. They are nourishing, relaxing, and rejuvenating. On the contrary, if the person is chilled, weak, and short of breath, I might recommend a warming or drying tonic that would help maintain a healthy water balance by preventing diarrhea and excess sweating. For example, sage or schizandra tea works for this.

If you suffer from menopausal hot flashes, chronic thirst, fevers, or diabetes, you may feel on fire or experience night sweats. The imbalance may be related to stress, inflammation, or hormonal tidal waves that temporarily disturb energy, blood production, and metabolism. You will likely benefit from a cooling, moistening, blood-enhancing tonic such as the Chinese patent remedy Liu Wei Di Huang Wan or a variation called Nine Flavor Tea pills from

Health Concerns. East Earth Trade Winds sells Recovery (White Turtle) Tabs and fo-ti pills, among others, that ensure moisture balance and energy resilience. Such Chinese formulas help the body to maintain normal water balance so that internal organs, especially the liver and kidney, are protected from stress.

Often yin-building (moisturizing) formulas combine balancing herbs along with rehmannia, a fortifying blood-enhancing herb. The pills are often recommended for chronic dry or sore throat, insomnia, facial flushing, hot sensation in soles and palms, blurry vision, ringing in the ears, dizziness, and in some cases sexual impotence. Excess sweating is reduced because the formulas reduce inflammation and stress.

Note: it is rejuvenating for hair and skin to follow a course of treatment of up to one month of these moisturizing pills. Use a larger than normal dose of 15 pills of the Chinese patent remedy or 5 pills of Nine Flavor Tea twice daily until you feel renewed and refreshed. Caution: as with any moisturizing formula, avoid using it during colds and flu because it increases mucus.

Fragrance Beauty

Fragrance is more than an indicator of symptoms. It announces your presence and creates an allure. It can also be used to brighten your mood, clear your senses, and settle your nerves. Here is how you can use your knowledge of the Chinese Five Elements. Do you need to gear up for an important event? Fragrance is subtle, but its effects run deep. Add a few drops of an essential oil to the final rinse after a shampoo or add some to your handwashed underclothes. Add an essential oil to water and spray it on anytime with an atomizer. You will feel the difference.

To spark high energy for a performance or public appearance, use a fragrance that is slightly bitter, smoky, or burnt-smelling to stimulate the heart, chest, and circulation, for example, myrrh. You might also substitute a bitter, pungent stimulant to help yourself to stop smoking (an inflammatory habit). Familiar bitter fragrances include cardamom, sage, rosemary, thyme, clove, and evergreen. Spray them on with an atomizer or add them to an energizing bath. To sooth rough, red skin and help prevent broken capillaries, Georgette Klinger makes a wonderful pure rose water that comes in an atomizer. I also like a cooling chamomile tea, which I keep in the refrigerator.

To soothe first-date nerves for yourself or a lover, use a heavy, grounding, and satisfying fragrance such as magnolia, gardenia, nutmeg, or apple. You will find a friend in apple blossoms. Research has shown that green apple and apple blossom aromas quiet anxiety.

To enhance courage and endurance, use a spicy, salty, or oceanic fragrance to strengthen your Water Element. The wide expanse of the ocean deepens breath and relaxes the mind. Fragrance is very individual. One person told me that the perfume Canoe was calming because it reminded him of sailing. Where do you want to be? What do you want to do? Choose a fragrance that takes you there.

If you need more creativity and personal vision, choose a fragrance that suggests new beginnings and the Wood Element. I enjoy the freshness of cucumber and mint, or an aroma that reminds me of mountains or sky. When I miss traveling or yearn for the exotic, I use Asian incense. Chinese incense is often cooling and energizing. Heady East Indian jute sticks made in Pondicherry or Tibetan healing incense that contains as many as 25 or more herbs, spices, and evergreens lift me out of the everyday into a broader world.

Herbal Extracts and Vinegars

It is fun to make your own beauty products. I have been doing it since childhood. Any herb can be made into a liquid extract or oil within three weeks. You might store them in attractive wine bottles and give them as gifts. The choice of herbs depends on your tastes and special needs.

Basic Recipes for External Use Only

I never measure; it's more fun to make things intuitively. However, this rough guide can get you started. If you are making an extract with spirits, use at least 1 ounce of raw or dried herbs per pint of liquid. You might use pure rubbing alcohol, vinegar, witch hazel, or other mediums that draw out the herbal essence and aroma.

The difference among these three is that alcohol makes a powerful extract. It takes less time to ripen and the aroma is stronger. Witch hazel is less drying and irritating to skin and scalp than alcohol. Vinegar works best for bath preparations that are deeply purifying. Its natural sour and astringent nature drains toxins from the body. With overuse, it might lower energy. Use a vinegar bath no more than once a week or three days consecutively. You might add pungent rosemary or clove to increase vinegar's stimulant qualities.

If the extract bottle's appearance is important, you might use some of the whole herb—leaves, stems, and berries. For 1 liter of 80–100 proof alcohol, add just enough loose herbs to make an attractive bottle. If you are interested more in the aroma of the liquid than the appearance, you can fill the bottle with up to 1 inch of powdered herbs, then fill the bottle with spirits leaving room at the top in order to let the herbs expand over time.

Steep liquid extracts in an airtight glass container in a cool, dark place for two or more weeks. You may occasionally gently turn the container to allow the ingredients to blend. It is not really necessary to change anything until you are ready to strain the ingredients.

On that day, sniff the mixture to decide if it's ready. It will seem stronger in the bottle than it will in your bathtub or as an after-bath splash. When you are satisfied with the results, strain the mixture through cheesecloth into your decanter or bottle and reseal. I have never kept such extracts long enough to judge the optimal shelf life.

Pour your creations into baths. Spray them on anything. If you use alcohol, avoid sensitive areas of the body. Use fragrances according to your energy needs and the Five Elements. For example, you might use cedarwood, lavender, or sandalwood extract to refresh the air during hot and muggy weather. The following recipes use kitchen herbs as fragrant medicines.

Egyptian Oils for Medicines and Beauty

Scrolls and fragments of papyrus found in the temple of Rameses II at Thebes were for the benefit of the medical profession—the wise men and priests who were skilled in the care of mind and body. However, everyone in villages knew the folklore of herbs that were used in a wide variety of ways. They were taken internally, applied as bandages and poultices, massaged into the skin, or given for inhalation. Aromatherapy and the use of fragrance in facial steam treatments and baths were widely used by all.

Aromatic oils were a practical medium used by early Egyptians and later Greeks for administering fragrance medicinally. Unfortunately, most Egyptologists are not herbalists. I will translate some of their findings for our use as beauty/health potions.

When making the following oils, try to use fresh herbs whenever possible. You should experiment with a small quantity of herbs and oil the first time you try this. For example, use one handful of fresh leaves (or myrrh gum) per small bottle (8.5 fluid ounces of olive oil). Other neutral oils you might use are walnut, sunflower, canola, or grapeseed oil. Crush the herb to release the fragrance and place it in oil for one month. Keep the bottle airtight in a dark, cool place. To make a stronger fragrance, steep the leaves in oil for three weeks, strain the oil, then add fresh herbs to the fragrant oil for another two weeks.

Basil oil was often used as a perfume and medicine. Dioscorides described its use for female complaints such as regulating menstruation. It is said to treat depression and anxiety. Energetically speaking, basil is diaphoretic: it increases sweating. That could make it strengthening for weak people who tend towards chills or diarrhea. Basil may also be an invigorating massage oil for timid people with a sallow or pale complexion.

Celery oil has a powerful scent. Leaves of wild celery were used as garlands for mummies in the 20th dynasty. The aromatic fragrance of celery oil is not as desirable as the anti-inflammatory effects the oil has on arthritic joints. Use olive or sunflower oil and celery seeds to make the oil and massage it into painful swollen joints.

Chamomile oil was described by Dioscorides in *On Medical Matters* to be used like radish oil to "cleanse scabrities bout the face." It was used in Egypt as an insect repellent and in mummification. Most of us know chamomile tea for indigestion. It also cools the skin and helps prevent irritation. Georgette Klinger uses the flowers to make a rich moisture cream that is suitable for rosacea or a ruddy complexion. If you make your own chamomile oil, use a cooling base such as sunflower oil and add dried Hungarian chamomile flowers, which are the most fragrant.

Cinnamon oil raises the body temperature and stimulates blood circulation and nervous excitability as it counters fatigue. It is also antibacterial. Cinnamon, myrrh, and juniper were widely used in mummification to prevent spoilage. I would use cinnamon oil during cold harsh weather as a foot massage oil or as a scalp massage for thinning hair. Use raw (not flavored) sesame oil and cinnamon powder to make the oil. Do not leave it on the skin for a long time because it can become too heating.

Cumin and dill oil are both mentioned as cooling pain remedies for headaches and menstrual problems. They have a refreshing, slightly bitter aroma when applied externally. You might use a handful of cumin seeds, dill flowers, and dried roses in safflower oil to make a fragrant massage remedy for treating an anxious headache or migraine.

Fenugreek means Greek hay. The seeds sprouted in water treat fevers and stomach ailments. Recent research has proven that the sprouts balance blood sugar in diabetes. Fenugreek tea, made by steeping the dried seeds in hot water, gives your entire body a pungent aroma. It is recommended in Asian medicine for asthma and sexual impotence because it is warming, stimulating, and diaphoretic. Lise Manniche describes an Egyptian medical text where fenugreek (hemayt) is the sole ingredient in an oil made by boiling the seeds in water to make a paste that "transformed an old man into a young man." Skin rubbed with it was left "beautiful without any blemishes. It is a million times efficient." This may describe not only a pungent complexion remedy but the world's first spread-on Viagra!

Marjoram oil cools sexual ardor. But be careful who you cool. A friend today might be a lover tomorrow. The ancient Greeks applied the oil to hemorrhoids to ease pain and to the female vulva to ease menstrual discomfort and bring on the period. The herb is a vasodilator useful for high blood pressure. In Chapter 9, I recommend oregano oil, similar to marjoram, as a scalp massage for thinning hair.

A Quick Fix for Eliminating Body Odors

Most odors can be eliminated with proper internal cleansing. I prefer drinking aloe vera gel to reduce poisons and bad breath because it is cooling, soothing, and relaxing. To reduce acidity, drink ½ cup or more of aloe vera gel daily. A twist of lemon or a drop of essential mint oil is optional. I prefer plain aloe's fresh high desert flavor.

Homeopathic silicea 30C can also be added to aloe and water. It works fast without any fuss and is inexpensive. Make sure to use homeopathic silicea between meals or on an empty stomach. Otherwise, it might diffuse digestive acids or give you heartburn.

At night, soak for five minutes in a tub of warm water to which you have added one cup of baking soda and ¼ cup of sea salt. It "brightens" your complexion and removes odor.

Especially for Men

Professional men (and women) who think and worry constantly get overheated. The curative quality of aloe vera gel helps soothe inflammation throughout the nervous system, including the brain. Ayurvedic herbalists recommend putting aloe gel inside the nose with a Q-tip in order to heal dry nasal tissue. It is also said to prevent red eyes, thinning hair, and bad breath from anxiety and anger. Bad breath comes partly from nasal and lung dryness as we exhale. Aloe in the nose and swallowed reduces dryness, burning, and odors.

Lola's Way

Do you feel like a rose, a peach, white linen, a sea mist, or an evergreen? What scent do you use and for what occasion? Do you have a signature fragrance, a scent that represents you? This section will free your creativity to use fragrance as an energetic tool.

We will associate colors with fragrance types. That sort of correspondence was established as a fundamental principle of ancient Chinese medicine nearly 5000 years ago in the *Huang Ti Nei Jing Su Wen* (the classic book of internal medicine attributed to Huang Ti, the yellow emperor). Ancient Chinese doctors who described the energetic forces that empower life believed that certain sounds, colors, flavors, and fragrances were related. For our experiment in personal alchemy, we are going to associate colors and fragrances according to their *energetic* effects upon us and others.

Warm Colors and Fragrances

Fragrances that seem pungent and have names such as rose, red door, rascal, or flame can be considered warm like the color red. Fragrances that are sweet in nature such as magnolia or honeysuckle can be associated with warm earth colors: yellow, orange, or gold.

Cool Colors and Fragrances

Fragrances that are dry, crisp, airy, and light—with names such as crystal, satin, white lace, or chantilly—can be white. Fragrances that are cool, dark, somber, heavy, rich, or smoky, and have names such as opium, can be black. Those which are spicy, stimulating, and exciting and have names such as stetson, leather, green grass, or rain can be green.

The fragrance flavors and qualities we will use for the following exercise are hot, sweet, dry or crisp, heavy or oily, and spicy. The associated colors are red and pink; yellow, orange-brown, and gold; white, cream, and beige; blue, black, and gray; and green. When in doubt, use your imagination.

Now look at your closet as well as your dressing table or bathroom cabinet. What do your color and fragrance choices say about you? Are you wearing bright clear colors with heavy, sedating fragrances? Are you dressed as somberly as a judge but smelling like bubblegum? Improve your energy and refocus your subliminal effects upon others by coordinating your colors and fragrances. The following chart illustrates the colors, fragrances, and positive emotions associated with the Chinese Five Element categories:

Color	Fragrance	Mood
Red	Hot	Joy
Yellow	Sweet	Mellow
White	Crisp, dry	Lofty, spiritual
Black or blue	Heavy	Dignified
Green	Woodsy	Enthusiastic

The order of colors is red, yellow, white, black or blue, and green, then back to red to make a circle. Choose a color, fragrance, and emotion group that you wish to express. For example: red, dramatic or hot, and joy. Then boost its charge by adding a color and fragrance accent from the group that precedes it. For example, to increase joy, enthusiasm or passion, wear the color red and a hot fragrance such as one called blaze. To build the flames higher, choose a few green accessories and dab on a woodsy scent somewhere warm enough to diffuse a smoldering flame. The point is to catch *you* on fire.

Style experts in later chapters recommend traditional clothing and makeup colors according to hair and skin tone. Use this mystical approach for your own program and keep it to yourself. The better part of magic is surprise. Use a fragrance to signal an emotion. Wear it someplace unexpected, such as on your hands and feet.

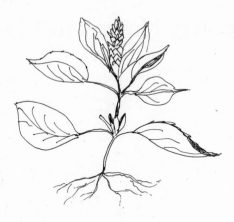

9

Pretty Hands and Feet

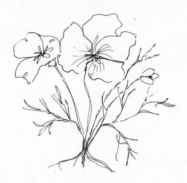

"When a lady lets her fingers softly linger in the palm
of a gentleman, what else does it say but, 'you have
my heart already.'"
—LOLA MONTEZ

Lola was right: you reveal your heart when you offer your hand. A nervous person may sit on her hands to keep them from trembling. Someone hot-tempered may wave them about in an argument. A lover's caress is the heart's message. In traditional Chinese medicine, the palms are linked with acupuncture meridians leading to the heart and pericardium, the protective sac that surrounds it. Skin discolorations, tingling sensations, and hot or cold palms reveal vitality and circulation. People who are warm-hearted may have cold hands when physically weak. Someone with a high-stress lifestyle might have hot, purple hands from poor circulation and dehydration.

Feet also indicate vitality. People with cold feet may or may not lack courage, but according to TCM they lack stamina. Cold feet can accompany diarrhea, backache, low sexual energy, or menstrual irregularities. One TCM imbalance, signaled by ice cold feet, is described as "cold uterus" and indicates functional infertility. We can adjust body temperature with diet, herbs, exercise, and treatments of hands and feet.

Your Energy and Ting Points

Most people want to improve the dryness, skin spots, brittle nails, or painful joints on their hands and feet. Most beauty shops offer treatments, including beautifying soaks and scrubs during manicures and pedicures. Have you ever relaxed to the point of falling asleep during a treatment? Hands and feet play an important role in maintaining energy and body temperature.

Near the cuticle on fingernails and toenails you can locate your *ting points* (the endings of acupuncture meridians) which, when punctured, lower internal temperature. *Ting* points are like the water spigots for a sprinkler system on your lawn. If the spigots are clogged, water builds up in the pipes and might explode. Something like that can also happen in the body. Here are two examples.

The summer of 2001, Korey Stringer, a 6'4", 335-pound 27-year-old right tackle for the Minnesota Vikings football team suddenly died of heat exhaustion during practice. He was wearing his full uniform. The temperature in the field was 90 degrees. His internal temperature, measured in the hospital, was 108 degrees. I was particularly saddened to realize how easily he might have been saved with traditional Chinese medicine.

Once in a beautiful northern Thai jungle near Chiang Mei, I was traveling by elephant along with a small group of friends from Bangkok. The heat was intense as we loped along, visiting local tribes who originated from China and Tibet. Teak trees grew high with broad shiny leaves. Rice patties stretched into long black mud grooves. When we stopped to rest under a grass awning, a young Thai student fainted and began to turn an odd color. I punctured the ting points of each finger and toe, letting a drop of blood escape. In an instant, she revived and was fine.

Energy Balancing with Hands and Feet

Later in this chapter, you will learn about complexion-beautifying hand and foot soaks. Soaking affects your energy because of the acupuncture meridians located at the fingertips. If you have chronic headaches or hot flashes, add some organic lemon juice to warm water when soaking hands and feet. Vitamin C and essential oils in the lemon feel cooling and comforting.

What's Hot Quickly Ripens

Most health experts believe that aging, emotional stress, and certain illnesses are increased by internal inflammation. The face may mirror the soul, but hands and feet reveal the battle between stress and vitality, especially the health of internal organs and blood circulation. As you discover beauty treatments to make your hands and feet more seductive, you can look for potential health problems. Here are some things to notice.

Color and Shape

Are the tips of your fingers or toes dark or discolored?
Are they swollen?
Do you experience burning pain in your fingers or toes?

Swelling, redness or discolorations, pain, or numbness in hands and feet can result from inflammatory conditions, sometimes leading to lumbago, sciatica, arthritis, and gout. We will touch on arthritis in a later chapter. Water pills used to reduce hypertension and aspirin both reduce uric acid excretion. This means the aspirin you are taking to help your heart may be increasing your risk of gout, kidney stones, and bleeding ulcers! Here are some ways to reduce excess-acid pain.

Increase Bitter, Cleansing Greens, and Natural Liver Cleansers

Inflammatory pain and swelling in fingers and toes can be improved by increasing your intake of cleansing bitter salad greens like chicory, watercress, dandelion, endive, and zucchini; high sodium foods such as celery, okra, and raw goat whey or Bernard Jensen's Capra Whey Powder. Homeopathic natrum sulphate 6x and natrum phosphate 6x strength, both cleansing forms of natural sodium (not table salt) reduce, respectively, water retention, nausea, and constipation as well as excess acid conditions, including joint pain and swelling, discomfort from stomach ulcers, or itchy, red complexion bumps. You can head off an acid attack by adding 10 pills of each remedy per quart of water. Sip it as often as every 15 minutes between meals until everything cools down. Also see amla on page 125. Some medical sources recommend drinking enough water daily to make two quarts of urine!

If you reduce uric acid naturally with homeopathic remedies and alkalinizing, diuretic foods, your joints will look more slender and graceful. Joint redness, swelling, stiffness, and pain can be reduced. You will suffer less from anxiety and eczema.

Circulation

Is the skin on your palms or soles dry and cracked?
Do your hands and feet tingle or feel numb?
Are your hands and feet always cold or wet?
Are they stiff every morning?

What feels better for them, hot water or ice?
Do you get leg or foot cramps or drawing pains?

Poor circulation can result from heart or adrenal irregularities, high cholesterol, and emotional upsets. These are frequent problems of stress aggravated by stimulants and caffeine.

Avoid Creating Problems

I have an elegant woman friend, an artist and free spirit, who received synthetic testosterone shots from her doctor to improve (she thought) her sex life—a bad idea. She then developed uterine fibroids. I noticed that her fingertips were alarmingly purple, a sign of poor circulation or, as Chinese doctors say, "stagnant blood." I recommended herbs to free circulation and dissolve fibroids and she got much better—uterus, fingertips, and all.

Circulation Herbs

If your stiff or sore joints feel better with an application of ice, the underlying imbalance is inflammatory (e.g., inflammatory arthritis). Use cooling foods and herbs such as bitter cleansing greens. Gotu kola tea or capsules are a cooling remedy recommended for tired legs and chronic fatigue from standing and sitting. Some people also use it for memory and mental clarity.

If joints and muscles feel better with warmth and massage, the underlying problem may be weakness and exhaustion. Use warming herbs. For example, hawthorn berry capsules strengthen the heart muscle to ease chest discomfort. One to two capsules taken after meals often prevents hand numbness. Avoid excess use if you have stomach ulcers or insomnia. Cinnamon and turmeric powder can be made into a traditional tea that eases shoulder stiffness and pain. A big pinch of each added to one cup of hot water makes shoulders, arms, and hands feel warmer. Avoid overuse during fevers.

Ginkgo improves blood circulation at the extremities, including hands and feet. If your hands are sallow or bluish, circulation is weak. You might consider taking one or more of these herbs.

Cracked Dry Skin

If your hands are dry and cracked like the bottom of a dried riverbed, circulation can be improved with homeopathic calcarea fluoride 6x, a remedy for weak internal organs that contribute to poor circulation, loose teeth, and weak bones. The dosage for most 6x strength homeopathic remedies is five times daily for chronic problems.

Cramps

The best homeopathic remedy I have found for acute and chronic leg and foot cramps is called Leg Cramp Relief, made by Natra-Bio in Ferndale, Washington. It contains liver-cleansing and liver-supporting ingredients such as homeopathic quinine sulphate, bitter apple, everlasting, calcium carbonate, lycopodium, magnesium, rhus toxicodendron, and copper. A few days of 3 pills daily between meals and 2 at bedtime prevents cramps. People with poor circulation, arthritis, and desk jobs can find relief if they use it on a regular basis.

Corns, Calluses, and Bunions

Ill-fitting shoes can aggravate corns and calluses. Bunions are big painful bumps on the joint of the big toe. Doctors say they are inherited or caused by pointed, high-heeled shoes that are too small. High heels throw the weight forward onto the toes, where they are crammed into narrow shoes. The medical solution is surgery. I once asked a Chinese doctor about bunions, and her response was, "Wear bigger shoes." That is also the medical consensus given by a panel of experts on www.webMD.com. However, there is a middle-road somewhere between wide loafers and the knife.

Bones swell and bend out of shape when bone rubs against bone. That happens every minute with your feet. There are 26 bones and 33 joints layered with an intertwining web of 126 muscles, ligaments, and nerves in the foot. The impact of every step exerts tremendous force upon the feet—about 50% greater than your body weight. The foot acts as a shock absorber and as a lever to propel the leg forward, and it serves to balance and adjust the body on uneven surfaces. Feet are always stamping, swerving, and twisting. It is not surprising, that about 75% of Americans experience foot pain.

One remedy to this is to provide a better cushion and support for your joints. Then less weight and direct impact will be exerted on the toes. Correct-fitting, low-heeled shoes are only part of the solution. To cushion joints, you need to increase foods and supplements that make joints slip and slide instead of grind against each other. Yucca, glucosomine sulphate, Asian sea cucumber, MSM (a form of sulphur), and mixed trace minerals insure better joint movement and freedom from pain.

Remedies for Joint Swelling and Pain

Joints need nourishment for natural protection from wear and tear. Typing and walking put extra stress on delicate joints. Several foods and supplements are helpful in preventing swollen, painful hands and feet.

Yucca grows wild in the American southwest and throughout Latin America, where it is eaten as a starch. You can find it dried or frozen in many supermarkets that carry tropical foods. I peel it and simmer it in water until soft, then add olive oil and fresh garlic for flavor. It's a tasty side dish that provides antioxidants and reduces cholesterol and excess sugar from the diet as it cushions the joints. Yucca has been used by American Indians as soap because it is slippery and sudsy. An antiinflammatory, it makes joints glide instead of grind. I have advised people with enlarged joints, especially knees and ankles, to take as many as 12–16 capsules daily.

Glucosomine sulphate and MSM are health-food store products recommended to help reverse painful swollen joints. They furnish the nourishment necessary to keep cartilage young. I add MSM to many of my blood-building herbal brews that I cook in a crockpot to insure that they will be taken to the blood and liver to nourish joints, muscles, and tendons. We will look at recipes in detail later.

Sea cucumber (*Microchele nobilis*) is a sea creature that lies in low Asian waters. The tasteless, jelly-like dish is a delicacy in China and Japan. It is considered a potent healthful tonic medicine for weakness. Fine Chinese restaurants, such as Goody's on East Broadway in New York City's Chinatown, combine it with deer tendons as a traditional Chinese gourmet dish. It eases joint and tendon pain and inflammation because it is moistening and nourishing for bone marrow, bones, and cartilage.

You can find sea cucumbers—large, black, shrivelled, worm-like objects—dried or packaged frozen in most Chinese groceries. But don't try to cook it yourself. That takes days of painstaking soaking, cleaning, and preparation. Try it in a restaurant or take pills such as Sea Q, made by Health Concerns, which contains sea cucumber and sargassum seaweed. A dose of 4 pills twice daily is recommended as a general tonic and antiarthritic, antiinflammatory remedy. For men who are weak and dehydrated, the pills are said to improve impotence.

Bone Spurs

A fantastic Chinese patent remedy recommended for bone spurs (multiplicative growth of bone matrix, spondylitis, hypertrophic thoracic, or lumber vertebra) and arthritic swelling is called Kang Gu Zeng Sheng Pian. Clients have told me that it significantly reduced bone spur and foot discomfort with one bottle. In most cases, 6 pills three times daily is recommended for one to three months and up to half a year in order to "replenish loin and kidney, strengthen muscles and bones, and increase blood circulation."

The pills contain blood-enhancing herbs and adrenal tonics, including rehmannia, cistanchis, and epimedium. It goes to show that bone is an outgrowth of marrow, blood, and kidney/adrenal energy. Rehmannia, a moistening blood tonic, revamps liver and kidney tissue. Cistanchis and epimedium, often recommended for sexual exhaustion, replenish testosterone and treat lower back weakness. (See Yin/Yang Sisters teas for energy and circulation comfort on page 233.)

Protect Your Hands, Feet, and Energy with Tonics

You may have to give up pointed high heels, but the real underlying causes of back, leg, and foot pain and deformity are adrenal exhaustion and improper nourishment aggravated by overwork, stress, caffeine, insomnia, illness, and excess weight—in a word, aging. To overcome those problems, use the stress-fighter herbs described in Chapter 3, the posture and foot exercises in Chapter 5, and the basic weight-loss diet in Chapter 6.

Nails

Are your fingernails fragile or splitting?
Do they turn downward at the tip?
Are your nails discolored or rough from a nail fungus?
Do your nails have ridges?
Do they have white spots on them?

A Chinese doctor may pinch your fingernails to see if the flesh underneath turns white and then pink. If the flesh remains pale, you have what they call blood deficiency and poor circulation. Once in Mexico I stayed with a family where the daughter had recently suffered a stroke. Obviously, with her circulation impaired, the flesh color under her nails was always stark white. Her hands felt like ice. Her speech improved along with her circulation and fingernail color as blood was able to move freely.

A fingernail with ridges or a down-turned tip can indicate damage from an injury or chemicals. However, Chinese herbalists equate fragile nails, teeth, and bones with under-nourishment and weakness. Imagine that your nails are an outgrowth of bone tissue and bone is an outgrowth of marrow. Blood-replenishing herbs such as (Chinese) Six Flavor Tea pills (Liu Wei Di Huang Wan) or (East Indian) Shilajet are quite helpful for beauty. They reduce stress as they moisturize internal organs and increase natural fluids.

If you tend to be thirsty or feel warm when everyone wears a sweater, cooling foods such as fresh sprouts, oatstraw tea, and nettle capsules will help you feel and look refreshed. They are high in natural silica, the mineral builder of bone, nails, and hair.

White spots on the nails show poor calcium absorption. It is useful to take a mineral supplement that includes trace elements necessary for calcium absorption. A good supplement would include calcium, magnesium, vitamin D, and zinc. Calcium is (poorly) absorbed in the large intestine. We require more calcium when under stress, and during the winter. Most people need at least 1000 mg of calcium and 500 mg of magnesium daily. For better absorption, take calcium along with something acidic such as orange juice. Another wonderful source of minerals is a homeopathic form of the 12 "tissue salts" called Bioplasma.

Nails: Care and Feeding

Nails, like hair and skin, are made of keratin, a fibrous protein, which is produced by cells located at the base of the nail underneath the cuticle. They are supposed to grow up to ½ inch every four months or more rapidly if you are between 18 and 28 years old or are pregnant. Dried beans, sprouts, organic eggs, yogurt, and seafood are especially nourishing sources of protein.

Horsetail (*Equisetum arvense*) looks like tall, stiff, green grass that grows along the highway on a riverbed. It is fibrous from silica, which makes it feel smooth like glass. Unless you recognize it in the wild, it is best to take health-food store capsules of horsetail that has been picked during the spring when its silica content is high. Horsetail picked later in the year may be irritating to the kidneys. For strong nails, drink at least three cups daily of horsetail tea between meals.

Fungus

Brigitte Mars in her netlibrary book, *Herbs for Hair, Skin and Nails,* advises to avoid trimming the cuticle because it seals the skin between the nail and underneath. Cut or cracked cuticles risks infection. To treat nail fungus, she recommends soaking nails in 7 drops of essential bay oil in a pan of warm water. Bay leaf is antifungal, antiseptic, and stimulating. I prefer applying Australian tea tree oil with a Q-tip to treat nail fungus, which works in two days or less.

Hand and Foot Soaks

For improving brittle nails, soak them in a glass container with 5 drops of essential oil of lemon along with 3 tablespoons of one of the following nourishing oils: flaxseed, olive, sesame, or wheat germ oil for one half hour daily. Lemon oil is a source of vitamin C that improves nail color and texture. After the soak, rinse your hands and buff each nail with chamois for a minute or until the color underneath the nail is bright red.

If bones and muscles ache from fatigue or arthritis, soak them in Epsom Salts (magnesium sulfate). Epso-Pine, a combination of magnesium sulfate, balsam, eucalyptus, and pine needle oils and blue and yellow dyes, is made by Majestic Drug Company.

I use 20 drops to 1 teaspoon of an essential oil mixed with hot water as a soak. Rosemary is stimulating. Oregano is very relaxing. Spruce and pine are refreshing. Add ginger powder to hot water for a foot soak that makes you perspire. Ginger is a warming stimulant for cold feet and hands.

Origins makes Sole Searcher, an exfoliant described as a "smoothing foot scrub," which contains finely ground lava stone, alcohol, and a number of herbs such as nettle, sandalwood, pine, lemon rind, peppermint, and nutmeg. It and Origins Foot Rest, a soothing foot soak, make a nice gift for someone who stands all day or wears high heels.

Once a week, give your hands and feet a beauty shock treatment by increasing the oxygen in your skin. Oxygen in our cells helps prevent aging, drying, infections, and rashes. Georgette Klinger's Oxygen products get their boost from hydrogen peroxide, which contains an extra molecule of oxygen. Give hands and feet a facial with Georgette Klinger's creamy Moisture Recovery Dry Skin Mask or Oxygen Mask followed by Advanced Oxygen Moisturizer. Their ingredients, energizing vitamins, and antioxidants increase skin elasticity and are deeply nourishing—a pleasure to use.

Massage

A chapter on hands and feet cannot be complete without a section for Chinese massage. Special acupuncture points located on the hands, feet, nose, and ears reflect the circulation and energy of the entire body. Some acupuncturists specialize on those areas of treatment. If you want to ease circulation in arms, chest, heart, lungs, and intestines, then massage your hands. If you feel depressed, soak your hands in warms water and essential oil of lavender, or chamomile; if agitated, use rose oil then gently massage your hands.

Sensitive areas on the soles of the feet are related to the kidneys, digestion, sexual organs, and back or leg pain. If you have hypertension, soak your feet in warm water and oil of oregano and massage briskly especially around and between the toes. The area between the toes relates to the head and eyes so that massaging there helps to ease tension. Oregano, taken internally as a tea or essential oil, lowers blood pressure by dilating blood vessels. Used in massage, it brings blood and oxygen to the skin.

To heighten sexual pleasure, massage feet with a few drops of warm sesame oil (calming) to which you have added rosemary or sage oil, which are adrenal stimulants. Their bracing aroma is stimulating. Essential oil of rosemary, sage, ginger, or mustard are helpful for fatigue, backache, and sexual weakness when applied to the feet. Use heating stimulants such as these sparingly to avoid headache and dizziness.

Applying stronger pressure to the center of the palm and the soles of the feet (underneath the instep) is relaxing because it encourages muscle tension to move toward the extremities. Anxiety, fright, and irritability can be calmed by massaging along the line on the inside of your wrist, where the hand joins the arm. Push that line deeply with the thumb of your opposite hand just before an audition or difficult performance to take a deeper, quieter breath.

For pretty feet that feel no pain, while sitting in your bathtub put a handful of Epsom salts onto your washcloth and scrub your feet. Origins Salt Scrub adds soy oil to moisturize and eliminate dead skin during a shower.

Shoe Heaven: The Proper Fit

Most of us buy shoes for appearance and pay attention to fit only after it starts to hurt. For expert advice, I called Sharlot Batton, owner of Montana Boot, who splits her time between her Soho, New York, studio and 200-acre ranch a few miles out of Whitefish, Montana. That morning in early August, she was harvesting lavender from her organic garden. She and her mother stay close to the land despite their movie star neighbors in nearby mountains. She told me, "In Winifred near the center of Montana, I can see moose and deer out my door."

An attractive blonde who can wield a cobbler's mallet, she has made stage shoes for over 50 Broadway shows. In her spare time, she makes great custom-made leather cowboy and cowgirl boots. I asked Sharlot, who has taught footwear patternmaking, design, and construction at the Fashion Institute of Technology for over 15 years, how shoes ought to fit. With her usual wry humor she replied, "Singers want them too big, dancers want them too small, actors want them pretty and will wear the boxes if they think they look good. Designing shoes for the stage is always a crapshoot with the actor, designer, director, and wardrobe supervisor (and the janitor) thinking they have to have something to say about the shoes. So I try to hit it somewhere in the middle so the wearer is comfortable and the shoes do what they need to do—work on a raked stage, swing from the rafters, or do a quick change."

That seems like a happy balance for us all to reach—foot comfort, beauty, and practicality. Foot doctors advise against shoes that cramp your toes or raise heels more than ½ inch.

Beauty Treatments for Hands and Feet

Lola Montez, in *The Arts of Beauty,* describes Spanish and French women who are in the habit of sleeping in gloves that are lined with a kind of pomade made from soft soap, salad oil, and mutton tallow to improve complexion. That's a lot of work for a sticky mess! You couldn't answer the phone or an e-mail wearing those gloves. For chapped hands, Lola made a wash from 3 ounces each of lemon juice and white wine vinegar and ½ a pint of white brandy. Some modern hand creams are also a problem. Alcohol, used in most perfumes, is drying and does not improve general health. Some over-the-counter products use inexpensive ingredients that degrade as they age, such as laurel sulphate which turns into formaldehyde.

If you can afford it, pamper yourself with a professional treatment. Here are examples from each coast. Halfway between New York and New England is Saratoga Springs, New York. Known for elegant country homes of steel barons such as the Whitneys, the town comes equipped with a world-class racetrack and a summer concert season.

Natalie Naigles operates Saratoga Skin Center in the Arcade Building on Broadway and swears by Dr. Hauschska's products. Natalie combines deep connective tissue massage with foot and leg treatments to make leg cellulite feel unwelcome. She uses Dr. Hauschska's rosemary oil, Rosemary Foot Balm, and St. John's Wort Foot Cream (Happy Feet).

On the west coast, a two-hour drive from Los Angeles is a private 56-acre spa and Hollywood celebrity hideout called Two Bunch Palms in sleepy little Desert Hot Springs, California. At the spa you pay a lot to dress casually, eat veggie cold cuts, and forget your stressful superstar status.

Two Bunch Palms massage therapists use everything from mud, clay, seaweed, herbs, and essential oils to sound and color therapy in order to soothe and beautify body and mind. Aqua reflexology gives you a stimulating foot massage in your private mineral water pool. You can also have a paraffin wax treatment for hands and feet. Because wax is airtight, it moisturizes and softens the skin. Two Bunch Palms offers aromatherapy manicure and pedicure treatments that feature a soak in mineral salts followed by a warm wrap and massage.

A Quick Fix for Nervous Tension

Choose a time when you might rest with your feet up or take a nap after this treatment. The flesh of our palms and soles is especially absorbent and reacts quickly to natural treatments.

Soak your hands and feet in hot water, Epsom salts (high in magnesium), and one of the following essential oils: lavender, rosemary, or lemon. For every quart of water use ¼ cup of Epsom Salts and 10 drops of the oil. Lavender's spicy aroma stimulates circulation and has been recommended to improve depression. Rosemary is stimulating for weak leg muscles. Lemon is refreshing for burning or red hands and feet.

After soaking for 20 minutes, use one of the following oils for a hand and foot massage: sesame or walnut oil (warming) are useful for insomnia and anxiety; sunflower, olive, or safflower (cooling) are useful for weight loss and overheated conditions. Press hard between the webs of fingers and toes and on tops and bottoms of hands and feet. Massage wrists, ankles, knuckles, and toes by gently twisting the skin as though you were tightening a jar lid.

Put on clean white cotton gloves and socks for 15 minutes as you lie flat with your legs propped against a wall. Then rinse with warm water. For menopausal women, I recommend applying Georgette Klinger's Prime Time Rebalancing Cream as a final step.

If you are still hyperactive after this treatment, cleanse your blood of impurities that might lead to painful joints by snacking on celery, watercress, parsley, carrots, and raw zucchini squash.

Products To Avoid

Dibutylphthalate, or DBP, used to be found in many popular brands of nail polishes, top coats, and hardeners. By now, the ingredients may have changed; read the labels.

DBP is used to help nail polish form an even film as it dries, to keep products blended and evenly consistent, and as an ingredient to help cosmetics penetrate the skin. According to a report made by the Center for the Evaluation of Risks to Human Reproduction in Alexandria, Virginia, DBP is particularly damaging to the male reproductive system, with effects ranging from reduced sperm counts to testicular atrophy. The highest quantity of DBP has been found among reproductive-aged women. Nail products that do not contain DBP include L'Oreal Paris Jet-Set Quick Dry Enamel, Revlon Nail Enamel, and Garden Botanika Natural Color Nail Color.

Especially for Men

Nylon socks do not allow the feet to breathe. Try natural silk, cotton, wool, and hemp socks. Gentlemen used to go to barber shops for a shave and haircut. Why not have "Guy Shops"—salons of men grooming men that provide relaxing massage, facials, hair and scalp treatments, and pedicures? A pedicure and manicure can reduce stress and improve performance as well as looks. According to health expert Dr. Bernard Jensen, "massaging the feet improves blood flow in the brain."

Lola's Way

In *The Arts of Beauty* Lola Montez wrote, "A beautiful hand performs a great mission in the life of a belle. Indeed, the hand has a language of its own, which is often most intelligible when the tongue and every other part of the human body is compelled to be mute." Everyone—not just massage therapists—can heal with their hands. A sympathetic or tender laying on of hands can comfort or entice a loved one. Massage their hands to reduce typing (or heart and chest) stress. Massage their feet to ease backache and to warm sexual interest. You can use the above examples to create a home spa for you and loved ones. The comfort you create will make you very beautiful in their eyes.

Part Three covers other aspects of your beauty that give pleasure without saying a word—your hair, eyes, complexion, and good taste in clothes, colors, and style. To increase the sensual bouquet you offer yourself and others, I include a chapter on the captivating powers of the voice.

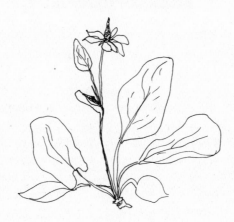

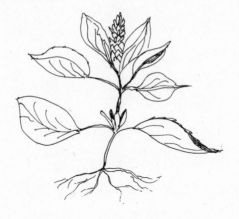

PART THREE

Beautiful You

"Now is the time to lay the foundations of power
and mastery for the future."
—*The I Ching or Book of Changes: Wei Chi*
(Before Completion).

10

Sexy Hair Shines from Within

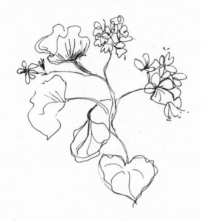

"Hair left to take care of itself will avenge itself
by making its possessor either common looking,
or a monster of ugliness."
—LOLA MONTEZ

Our hair can be a constant irritation in more ways than one. In *The Arts of Beauty,* Lola described nineteenth-century hair products that damaged appearance and poisoned users. Today's commercial brands contain chemicals that few people would gladly ingest. Oddly, we consider our hair to be separate from our interior selves. On bad hair days, we wish it did not belong to us at all.

Asian health theory defines hair as an outgrowth of our blood and bone marrow. That makes perfect sense to someone who has lost hair as a result of chemotherapy. In the hair-loss section of this chapter, you will learn ways to enhance hair growth from the scalp to the ends. Here is a shocker: excess testosterone is dehydrating and can lead to hair loss. But not only men lose hair. Do you have bloodshot eyes, thirst, or menopausal dryness along with thinning hair? Everyone needs internal moisture enhanced by foods and herbs to nourish hair below the scalp. If you lack moisture and nourishment in your hair fiber, no amount of creams and conditioners can maintain its beauty. Hair fiber is made of keratin, an insoluble protein that contains high amounts of sulfur as cystine. Aging, stress, and junk foods starve hair so that it loses luster and eventually falls out.

How Nourished Is Your Hair?

Here is an experiment to check whether the protein and minerals in your hair are adequate. Add one scoop of a health-food store protein powder to a glass of half water and half pineapple or papaya juice. I prefer Capra Mineral Whey powder, which is made from goat's milk and distributed by Bernard Jensen Products. If within a few minutes after drinking the mixture your hair smells like the drink, then you lack adequate hair nutrients. The protein has gone to where it is needed to build hair, skin, and nails.

Hair Foods

Protein and Minerals

From the moment of conception, our body uses protein to manufacture cells for growth and maintenance of bone and tissue. The stomach breaks down complete proteins into amino acids, which are transported from the small intestine and intestinal wall to the blood stream.

Protein found in bee pollen, royal jelly, and goat whey comes complete with all the necessary amino acids and is easily absorbed. Pollen and royal jelly are pure plant proteins predigested by bees. Unfortunately they are damaged by air, heat, and time. Capra Mineral Whey Powder contains minerals that work together in optimal combinations such as calcium, magnesium, manganese, and phosphorus along with iron; copper and iron with zinc; and sodium with potassium. Sodium, potassium, and calcium work together to keep the body alkaline while they reduce fatigue, indigestion, constipation, ulcers, heart irregularities, and chronic joint pain. People who are allergic or lactose intolerant usually have no problem with goat dairy because it lacks casein.

Sulphur adds luster and body to hair. It also helps fight bacterial infections. According to Earl Mindell, author of the *Vitamin Bible,* sulphur helps maintain oxygen balance necessary for proper brain function. It works with B-complex vitamins for basic body metabolism and is part of tissue-building amino acids. Recommended sources of sulfur include dried beans, fish, eggs, cabbage, avocado, Brussels sprouts, carrots, cauliflower, chervil, chives, egg whites, horseradish, mustard greens, white onions, papaya (including the seeds, which can be made into a tea), parsley, and watercress.

Silicea (natural silicon) makes fiber such as skin and hair solid yet flexible. Silicea gives shape to plants like grass and horsetail herb. Internally, the mineral keeps tissues alkaline therefore healthy. Sprouts and cooked oatmeal and barley are high sources, which makes them remarkable foods for convalescence.

Homeopathic potassium (kali sulphuricum 6x) promotes normal sweating. It enhances oxygen in the cells for beautiful skin and hair. Homeopathic sulphur 6x is recommended for stubborn skin problems and itching; and homeopathic silica 6x for weak bones and hair, slow healing skin sores, fragile fingernails, and unpleasant body odors. For chronic fevers or other inflammation, a dose of homeopathic iron (ferrum phosphate 6x) will feel cooling and rejuvenating. You can add one dose (5 pills) of each to a glass of water and drink it between meals.

Teas for Great Hair

Oatstraw tea (silicea) sweetened with black cherry concentrate, a potent source of iron, is a revitalizing hair food. Simmer one handful of dried oatstraw herb in 1 quart of water for 20 minutes. You can keep this in the refrigerator for up to one week. Bernard Jensen's Black Cherry Concentrate is available in many health-food stores as well as from Bernard Jensen Products listed in the Annotated Resource Guide at the back of this book.

The moistening Chinese herb he shou wu (*Polygonum multiflorum*), normally recommended for enhancing blood and sexual fluids, also improves hair. Internal moisture prevents broken ends and dull, lifeless hair. He shou wu, which means "black-haired Mr. He," is often recommended for premature graying hair. It also treats dizziness, blurry vision, weak lower back muscles, and insomnia. An antiinflammatory, it has been used for reducing skin sores, goiters, constipation, cholesterol, and malarial fevers.

He shou wu should be simmered for 45 minutes to an hour in order to make a decoction. Use one handful of dried herb per quart of water in a ceramic-coated or glass (nonmetal) pot. A good dosage to start with is one or two cups per day between meals. Since he shou wu is moistening, it slows digestion or can cause diarrhea if overused. A sure indication that you need it is that your palms and soles feel too warm and your hair is prematurely gray. If you have chronic chills or a pale, moist tongue, indicating water retention or mucus in the digestive tract, cook a handful of dried he shou wu along with one Chinese ginseng root to strengthen digestion. Add a pinch of cinnamon powder per cup of he shou wu decoction to insure better absorption and blood circulation.

Hair Honey and Wine

The following recipes, adapted from the book *Chinese Medicated Diet,* used by doctors studying at Shanghai College of Traditional Chinese Medicine, are recommended to improve hair strength, luster, and bounce.

Berry Honey

You might add a spoonful of this special honey to sweeten tea. It is considered useful for premature gray hair, deafness, constipation, insomnia, forgetfulness, blood deficiency after illness, and for what the Chinese call premature senility. Most of us have it.

For berries use Chinese lycium fruit, mulberries, blackberries, or bing cherries. Most berries are moistening and blood-enhancing. Mulberry contains carotene, thiamine, riboflavin, vitamin C, tannin, and linoleic acid. Big, sweet, black bing cherries are also useful for arthritic pain.

Ingredients:
3 cups fresh or 2 cups dried berries
1 cup dried sliced he shou wu
1 cup raw honey

Add the berries and he shou wu into a crockpot and cover with enough water to fill the pot. Cook with low heat for up to 10 hours or until the mixture turns thick and sticky. Cool then strain the mixture. After it is cold, add the honey. Pour it into a glass container for storage. Dosage: 1 tablespoonful at a time, morning and evening, infused in a cup of warm but not hot water. Caution: avoid using too much of this mixture if you tend to have bloating or diarrhea.

Bright Hair Wine

There is a long, dizzy history of Chinese herbal liquors. The effects are convincing. One sip feels like a right to the jaw with a bitter/sweet aftertaste. Here is a recipe recommended to "warm the kidneys, replenish lungs, and cure dry cough." It refines skin texture and makes hair glossy.

Ingredients:
One big handful (20 g) each of the following blood-enhancing herbs:
    wolfberry (*Lycium chinense*); longan (*Arillus longan*); ligustrum
    (*Fructus ligustri lucidi*); rehmannia root (*Radix rehmanniae*);
    epimedium (*Herba Epimedii*); and dried mung beans

1–2 liters of spirits (vodka, vermouth, or brandy)

Optional walnut oil or ghee (clarified butter)

Dried black mission figs to taste

Many Chinese blood-increasing herbs are semisweet fruits. I have added dried figs, an excellent source of potassium, as a sweetener. Vodka is neutral tasting. If you like a sweeter brew, use vermouth. Epimedium is a warming adrenal tonic and aphrodisiac. The original recipe calls for 100 g of lard, apparently to "brighten" the skin. I think the recipe can stand without it. Otherwise, for richness, add ⅛ cup ghee or walnut oil instead of lard.

Soak the dried herbs and fruit for five minutes to remove dust. (I use a dash of potassium salt substitute and apple cider vinegar in water.) Collect the mixture into a piece of cheesecloth tied at the top with a string. Put them into an airtight glass jar along with the (optional) oil and enough liquor to cover them. The herbs will double in size during steeping. Steep the herbs in the sealed jar in a dark, cool place for one month. Check the flavor after one month. You can decant it then or leave in the herbs for a stronger flavor.

I recommend no more than one wine glass daily. People who are allergic to alcohol can slow cook the mixture in a crockpot for 10 hours. The dosage for the water extract is ¼ cup daily between meals.

Hair Supplements

Seaweeds

A daily supplement of mixed trace minerals may be safer and easier than eating cooked seaweed to get the same iodine and potassium. Many supplements offer balanced nutrition and have warnings about seaweed on the label. Dry hair needs iodine and potassium found in dulce and kelp. Their minerals improve hair, skin, teeth, and nails because they speed metabolism to make new cells. Kelp pills can help prevent mental dullness, weight gain, irregular periods, and low energy by stimulating the thyroid gland. Kelp is an important ingredient in some weight-loss pills.

However, kelp is stimulating for hyperthyroid conditions and can make some people feel crazed and insomniac. Lesser sources of iodine are pineapple, eggs, peanuts, lettuce, spinach, and green peppers. I do not recommend taking more than 500 micrograms (mcg) of iodine from kelp per day. Watch for side effects and reduce the dosage if you become too speedy. Potassium clears thinking by sending oxygen to the brain. It speeds cleansing and waste disposal by preventing edema (water retention). It reduces blood pressure and helps prevent allergies. Dulce yields 8060 mcg of potassium per 100 g;

kelp 5273 mcg. If you tend to be emotional or nervous, avoid using kelp or dulce daily.

Chinese Herbal Supplements

It is best to take hair supplements between meals. That way they do not interfere with digestion. A TCM-inspired line of hair products, including pills, shampoo, and a topical liquid for thinning hair, is called Shen Min. Shen Min hair nutrient pills made by Biotech for men and women provide concentrated he shou wu herb along with herbs designed to improve overall health. The men's Shen Min hair nutrient formula contains saw palmetto and isoflavones from soy to protect prostrate health. The women's Shen Min hair nutrients formula contains black cohosh for hormone balance, uva ursi and burdock for water retention, as well as ginkgo, silicea, and horse chestnut for improved circulation. The recommended dose for Shen Min hair nutrients for men or women is 1 pill twice daily. Usually at least four months of use is required to make a difference for hair condition, but you may feel improvements in energy almost immediately.

Another fine source of nutrients is in Hair, Skin, and Nails made by Shen Min. You can take 2 tablets twice daily between meals along with nettle tea.

Astra Essence herbal pills made by Health Concerns contains astragalus, ligustrum, he shou wu, lycium fruit, rehmannia, eucommia, cuscuta, Chinese ginseng, tang kuei, and cornus. Like other Chinese hair products, it contains blood-enhancing herbs combined with adrenal stimulants (eucommia, cornus, and ginseng) in order to improve vitality and circulation. Astra Essence is normally recommended for degenerative conditions and deterioration of brain function (such as Alzheimer's disease), vertigo, hearing loss, dizziness, and poor memory from blood and energy weakness. It strengthens immunity and speeds recovery from illness. It is especially useful after chemotherapy and radiotherapy as an overall tonic as well as for hair loss. The dosage is normally 3 tablets three times daily between meals. You will find instructions for ordering from Health Concerns in the Annotated Resource Guide.

Tien Ma Tou Tong Wan, one of the best-known Chinese patent remedies for healthy hair, is available online or from local Chinese herb shops in your area. It contains gastrodia, a nerve tonic; he shou wu; ligustrum; and schisandra. It is recommended to nourish blood and disperse "wind" or nervous agitation. Gastrodia (a.k.a. tien ma) is a nerve stabilizer used for tremors and spasms. The formula treats "mental uneasiness" and provides nutrition for the hair. Tien Ma Tou Tong Wan's indications include "dizziness, neurasthenia, mental depression, pain and numbness of extremities (hands and feet), as well as white hair and hair loss."

By studying this formula you can see that blood and nerve tonic herbs affect everything from mental clarity and motor skills to hair loss! The recommended dosage for Tien Ma Tou Tong Wan is 6 pills twice daily between meals. The same caution concerning moistening herbs applies to this and most other herbal hair beauty remedies: if digestion is poor, add digestive herbs during meals. If a moistening formula causes diarrhea, reduce the dosage and add Chinese ginseng.

Home Beauty Treatments

Nourishing East Indian Herbal Treatments

Ayurveda, the traditional medicine from India, uses foods, herbs, and oils to increase beauty, vitality, and awareness. Often an East Indian grocery will have many beauty remedies designed for home use. Many are deeply nourishing and rejuvenating. In that way, they profoundly affect the mind and emotions. Cool your hot head with one of these beautifying herbal treatments and reduce headaches and nervous insomnia. They include two of the most popular rejuvenating herbs from India used as teas as well as hair treatments. Remember, your scalp absorbs nutrients too.

Vitamin C in Amla

Amla (*Emblica officinalis*; *Euphorbiaceae*) is an East Indian sour cherry that is extremely high in vitamin C, yielding 3000 mg per fruit. The powder is recommended internally as a rejuvenating tonic especially for anemia, diabetes, gout, gastritis, colitis, hepatitis, osteoporosis, constipation, bilious liver, premature graying hair and hair loss, and general debility. The high vitamin C content rebuilds tissue and increases red blood cells. Amla cleanses breath, strengthens teeth and bones, and increases hair and fingernail growth. It is useful for people with rich diet habits and a large waistline, joint pains, and bleeding gums.

Amla powder, made into a thick paste by adding warm water, can be applied as a scalp and hair pack to cool the head and build hair strength at the root. Leave it on covered with a plastic cap for at least two hours. It does not color the hair, but its vitamin C content feels invigorating and healing.

Improve Hair and Brain

Brahmi, sanskrit for gotu kola, is a famous East Indian herb for improving memory. According to Hindu tradition, brahmi (*Hydrocotyle asiatica; Umbelliferae*) increases awareness of supreme reality—Brahman. It is a nervine for calming nervous disorders and is recommended for anxiety, epilepsy, senility, premature aging, hair loss, and chronic nervous skin conditions. It is said to increase intelligence and decrease the effects of aging while it strengthens immunity and adrenal energy. Used externally, gotu kola paste is used for skin conditions like psoriasis. Hesh Pharma, the Bombay company which makes both amla and brahmi hair powders, recommends a brahmi powder pack for "long dense black lustrous hair." It strengthens hair roots and stops premature graying. It can be used as a scalp massage to eliminate dandruff and "gives sound sleep." That alone may increase intelligence. Bravo!

Vatika made by Dabur is a hair oil suitable for scalp massage that is made with coconut oil enriched with henna, amla, brahmi, cooling skin-purifying neem leaves, and lemon essence. After leaving one of these rich oils on the scalp overnight you may want to retreat to a mountain top and mumble chants. You can make your own favorite hair tonic using essential oils, jojoba oil, and a little gotu kola tea. Massage it lightly into the scalp and brush it through for at least 100 strokes.

A Mud Treatment for Dandruff

Eczema, dandruff, or patches of dry skin prevent hair growth through clogged pores. Some men complain of ingrown hairs after shaving. This cleansing treatment for skin and scalp has two parts—a cleansing mud pack and a rinse. Once a week, pull out impurities and clear the pores by applying a pack of dead sea mud onto your scalp the same way you would on your face. Cover with a plastic cap and let it harden for at least two and up to three hours. Gently wash with warm water until the water is clear. Then if needed, use a very mild shampoo one time only and conditioner only on the hair ends, not the scalp.

Towel dry and gently massage the following honeysuckle/dandelion/tea tree oil rinse on to the scalp. You can make up lots of this mixture and keep it in the refrigerator for up to one week. Use it as often as you like to clear blemishes and clogged skin. Simmer a handful each of honeysuckle flowers and dandelion herb in 1 quart water for 30 minutes. Cool and strain it through cheesecloth. Add 10 drops of Australian Tea Tree Oil to the mixture in order to clear infections or allergies. Use this as a final rinse to gently massage into the scalp.

Herbs for Renewing Original Hair Color

He shou wu is the best-known Chinese herb for prevention of premature gray hair. It comes as a loose herb for cooking as a decoction as well as pills called Shou Wu Pien. The dosage for the pills is normally 5 pills three times daily between meals. If you have indigestion or bloating, use additional digestive herbs.

Nettle tea is strongly recommended by an actress friend of mine, Anne, who has regained her original color without using hair dye. She makes the tea daily by putting a handful each of dried nettle and oatstraw into a mason jar, filling it with water, and leaving it in the sun all day. The next day she drinks the liquid. Her general health has improved over a period of a year. Nettle, a blood cleanser, fights allergies and weakness. Her hair looks thick, shiny, and soft—a lovely natural dark golden blonde.

Herbal Hair Color Products

Teas

Chamomile, sage, and nettle teas are used traditionally as hair dyes mainly because they are good for the hair root and texture. Chamomile or turmeric powder slightly warms up a dull blonde color, while sage, thyme, and nettle drab down overly bright colors. If you want to use the raw herbs as a final rinse, make a large pot of tea in a nonmetal container. Strain it and store it in the refrigerator for no more than two days.

Health-Food Store Brands

Jason, Weleda, BioForce, and Origins all make natural shampoos that are full of herbs to increase luster and bounce. Their natural-looking semipermanent colors contain little or no ammonia. Natural hair colors shimmer from herbal and flower ingredients that neither irritate nor dry hair and scalp. They add subtle highlights. Aveda makes a temporary hair color shampoo that deposits natural color on the hair without damaging it. They have two shades: Blue Malva, useful for toning down brassy yellows and red shades, contains chamomile, eucalyptus, geranium, and mint; Chamomile, a warm yellow color, contains the flower for which it is named.

Weleda's hair and scalp products use extra mild ingredients, including soap derived from coconut oil. Their herbal ingredients give hair a subtle boost in highlights, but are not a dye. For children and adults with delicate hair, Weleda makes Calendula Shampoo, which is soothing to the skin. Rosemary Shampoo and Conditioner are suitable for oily hair and medium to dark color. They do not strip natural oils and keep hair neat and manageable. Lemon Balm Shampoo works well for dry and damaged hair. For added highlights, consider Chamomile Shampoo and Conditioner for fair hair and Henna Shampoo for auburn. Chestnut Shampoo is recommended for normal hair.

Henna

Powdered Henna leaves (*Lawsonia inermis*) can color gray hair but look best on dark hair. Henna is a shrub that grows in the Middle East, North Africa, and the East Indies, where most women have black hair. Fiery henna-red hair heralded my student days in Paris. For many, it represents a passing phase. Most forms of henna can be used only on hair that has not been color processed. However, Hennalucent, made by Ardell International (www. aiibeauty.com) has several shades of organic henna that can safely be applied to color-treated hair. The color is very difficult to remove because it penetrates the hair shaft. Neutral henna drabs brassy reds. It gives hair fiber strength, body, and luster. However, it is drying.

Letha's Herbal Hair Rinse

This feels marvelous! I sometimes drink the following brew as well as splash it on my hair as a final rinse after a shampoo. My recipe calls for Chinese herbs known to enrich blood and vitality—no chemicals or preservatives. This rinse works best with ash blonde or darker tones because it does not lighten hair and lends a beige or ashen cast.

The recipe includes a handful each of he shou wu, ligustrum, a piece of dong quai, rehmannia, and a handful of cistanche. These are all semisweet blood-enhancing Chinese herbs. Cistanche (rou cong rong) is a kidney tonic normally recommended for sexual weakness and lower back and knee pain. It moistens and is laxative for elderly or weak people who lack adequate fluids. A blood-enhancing tonic such as this recipe is recommended to improve blood quality and energy in order to prevent osteoporosis, chronic pain, and aging. To increase immunity, you might add a piece of ling zhi mushroom (ganoderma) to cook with the other herbs.

Add the herbs to a crockpot filled with water and cook over low heat for six hours or overnight. Strain it through cheesecloth and store it in the refrigerator for up to one week. The rinse will add bounce and shine as it softens stiff unmanageable hair. It feels soothing and relaxing because you are nourishing blood and bone marrow.

To use this brew as a semipermanent hair dye (for medium to dark hair) requires one more step. When the time comes to dye your hair, reheat the herbal mixture and add it instead of hot water to neutral or colored henna, black tea, or chamomile tea. Don't drink it if you add henna!

Hair Loss

Hair grows from the hair follicle at an average rate of a 1/2 inch per month. Each hair grows for two to six years, then rests and finally falls out. Periodically we have a new head of hair. Baldness often occurs when hair fails to grow through clogged pores. Hair loss is associated with genetic predisposition, aging, and levels of endocrine hormones. Excess testosterone causes facial hair and head hair loss in women, especially after menopause. Men with thick hair and flabby muscles may be lacking in testosterone.

Testosterone is produced by the coordinated efforts of the pituitary gland and testes in men and the pituitary gland and adrenal glands in women. When overstimulated from stress, fatigue, illness, caffeine, drugs, or other factors—including menopause—those glands overwork. Many people tend to feel nervous, insomniac, anxious, or hyper when fatigued. Those factors also produce the *effects* of excess testosterone whether or not hormones are involved: call it nervous exhaustion and dehydration. The resulting thirst, sweating, or excitability feels as though we are ready for fight or flight. This tension eventually dries body fluids that nourish hair and skin.

One way to avoid stress is *not* by taking a potentially dangerous drug. FDA-approved Minoxidil is used topically on the scalp and works by inhibiting naturally occurring hormones. However, a solution higher than 2% can cause birth defects. It improves hair growth only an estimated 10% of the time. Used twice daily, the drug costs in excess of $600 yearly. Its use must be continued if it is to work at all. Obviously, a better solution is necessary for people with thinning hair—according to best estimates nearly half of all adults in the United States by age forty.

Genetics are not everything. Unnatural hair loss in women often accompanies recovery from childbirth or debilitating illness. Other factors include poor circulation, a lack of certain minerals, hormonal factors, and skin problems such as eczema. If your tongue is pale and you feel short of breath, the first thing to do is to lift your energy and spirits. That will improve circulation.

Blood and Energy Deficiency-Related Hair Loss

Chinese women recovering from childbirth, exhaustion, or serious illness often take Buzhong Yi Qi Wan, which contains astragalus, licorice, tang kuei, cimicifuga, codonopsis, atractylodes, citrus peel, bupleurum, jujube, and ginger. Buzhong Yi Qi Wan is normally recommended for prolapsed internal organs, hemorrhoids, varicose veins, spotting or uterine bleeding, and chronic diarrhea from weakness. Using a tonic that "lifts" energy can get more blood and circulation up to your head. Healthy hair also needs L. cysteine, an amino acid. It is wise to take a full-spectrum amino acid combination such as that found in a whole food, royal jelly. Ginseng and Royal Jelly (extract capsules) is a famous longevity and beauty tonic used by generations.

Other useful Chinese herbs are so called "yin" tonics that increase nourishment and moisture. Shou Wu Pien pills (*Polygonum multiflori*) nourish the building blocks for hair, skin, and nails. I recommend using it along with ginkgo biloba, which increases circulation especially in the head and all extremities. For example, between meals you might take 5 pills of Shou Wu Pien and 2 capsules of ginkgo twice daily. Han lien cao (*Eclipta alba*) is another Chinese "yin" tonic sometimes used to promote new hair growth. Known as bhringraj in Sanskrit, the herb is cooling and moistening, therefore it is best used during hot weather. Otherwise, excess use may cause chills.

I have recommended han lien cao powder taken in empty capsules or with water after meals for people with thinning hair and visible inflammatory symptoms such as flushed appearance, night sweats, feverish feelings, hot flashes, or a dry reddish tongue and fast pulse. One young model was over-joyed. After using six capsules daily of han lien cao for one month, she saw tiny new hairs growing in her scalp where there had been balding.

Other blood-enhancing tonics that indirectly encourage new hair growth include the Chinese patent remedy Liu Wei Di Huang Wan, whose principle ingredient (*Rehmannia glutinosa*) is a yin tonic for liver and kidneys. Another blood tonic made by Health Concerns is Nine Flavor Tea pills, which contains rehmannia, dioscorea, poria, cornus, moutan, alisma, dendrobium, scrophu-laria, and ophiopogon. The formula covers a wide range of inflammatory and blood-deficiency problems, including chronic sore throat, oral sores, facial flushing, hot feeling soles of feet and palms, night sweats, menopausal inflam-mation, blurry vision, dizziness, tinnitus, and impotence that is related to stiff lower back muscles, blood deficiency, or nervousness.

For optimum protection against hair loss, men or women might use sev-eral of the above tonics at the same time between meals. For example, com-bine up to 6 pills of Buzhong Yi Qi Wan; 2 Ginseng and Royal Jelly capsules, 5 Shou Wu Pien pills, and 2 ginkgo capsules twice daily, at midafternoon and in the evening. If you need more energy, increase the dose of Ginseng and Royal Jelly. If the herbs feel too stimulating, increase the moistening Shou Wu Pien. If you continue to feel overheated or insomniac, use only Shou Wu Pien pills or Nine Flavor Tea pills. Eventually stress and inflammation symp-toms will stop.

Dandruff, Eczema, or Psoriasis-Related Hair Loss

Most people suffering from hair loss actually have chronic skin problems ranging from dry or itchy complexion and ingrown hairs to long-term skin diseases that require blood-cleansing complexion herbs in order to assure proper oxygen and blood circulation to the scalp. I recommend starting with a cleansing, low-fat diet of mainly fruits and vegetables. In addition, the fol-lowing skin cleansing herbs are in order.

Lien Chiao Pai Tu Pien, the Chinese patent remedy, and Skin Balance made by Health Concerns are discussed in the complexion chapter. Taking one of those between meals will help clear facial and scalp complexion. Healthy skin allows new hair roots to grow.

A good antidandruff shampoo will most likely contain salicylic acid, from willow, which is used for acne. One good brand is Herbal Essences Anti-Dandruff shampoo by Clairol, which also contains the Chinese herbs iris, chrysanthemum flower, and mulberry root for cooling skin inflammation. The Clairol Herbal Essences conditioner for dry scalp contains antibiotic honeysuckle flower along with soothing daisy and comfrey. They are a real herbal bath for your hair.

An Expert Tip for Brittle Ends

Here are two ways to prevent brittle ends. One elegant Italian stylist told me that his favorite natural bleaching treatment is to streak hair with lemon juice while sunning on the beach. Setting with curlers can break your ends. The gentlest way to curl hair is an old trick used during Civil War days. Cut a clean old shirt or handkerchief into strips that measure about 7 inches long and 4 inches wide (which can vary depending on your hair length). After washing and towel drying, take a bit of damp hair and lay it lengthwise in the cloth. Fold over the cloth to completely surround the hair in a long strip. Roll up the strip into a smooth curl and tie the two edges of the cloth at the top. Let the hair dry in the cloth-covered curl. When you remove the cloth, your hair will look as soft and wavy as Scarlett O'Hara's!

An Herbal Quick Fix for Healthy Hair and Scalp

Enjoy a 5-minute scalp massage with a few drops of one of the following: jojoba rosemary oil, oregano oil, tea tree oil, or Shen Min Topical liquid hair nutrients. Rosemary awakens the senses, stimulates energy, and warms the scalp. Oregano is relaxing and lowers blood pressure by dilating blood vessels. Tea tree oil clears the senses and prevents infection, yeast, dandruff, and ringworm. It acts as a stimulant for people who feel cloudy or heavy headed.

Topical, made by Shen Min, contains time-released soy protein and herbs, including nettle, saw palmetto, chamomile, and eucalyptus in order to stimulate follicle metabolism and inhibit free-radical binding. It increases peripheral blood circulation as it supplies nutrients, and has no unpleasant side effects.

Oils for Healthy Bounce and Shine

During hot weather or a trip to the tropics, avoid oily products that make hair sticky and limp. During cold weather or a skiing trip, seal in moisture with a richer hair treatment, including shampoo and scalp massage products. Lola Montez had coarse dark hair. In *The Arts of Beauty,* she praises a shampoo made with egg whites and rum that I am more tempted to drink as punch. The most important thing is the recipe contains no drying soap or alcohol. If you have oily skin and scalp it is all right to use some alcohol, but watch your diet to avoid trouble. Oily, spicy, and rich foods are congesting and clog pores. This chart summarizes essential oils suitable for scalp treatments and herbal shampoos.

> For blonde or fragile hair: oil of lemon and eucalyptus
> For dark hair or to reduce brassiness: oil of geranium, thyme, sage, or rosemary
> For eczema, psoriasis, warts, and dandruff: thyme oil
> For dandruff: oil of cedarwood, clary sage, lemon, patchouli, pine, rosemary, or a few drops of tea tree oil added to another essential oil (leave in overnight)

Hypoallergic Products
For An Especially Sensitive Scalp

Flowers and Spice and Everything Nice

Chemicals additives, alcohol, or perfumes tend to dry sensitive or blemished skin and scalp. The following major brands eliminate all irritating ingredients. Kiss My Face's Obsessively Natural Hair Care line combines essential oils and botanicals to create the rich vibrant feel of flowers and forests. Ingredients include chamomile, rosemary, lemon balm, nettle, and organic aloe. Their amusing names guide your selection: Big Body, SaHaira (of course, for dry hair), Whenever (for frequent shampoos), Miss Treated, Light Weight conditioner, Conditioned Response (for dry damaged hair), and Upper Management, a natural gel for fly-away hair. Imagine, some ingredients found in nonenlightened hair-setting gels are flammable!

Origins zesty hair products include Clear Head Mint Shampoo and Knot Free Finishing Rinse, which smells delicious with its peach, lemon, and peppermint fragrance. If your hair is straw dry, try Origins The Last Straw made rich with wheat protein, apricot and yarrow.

Ingredients from the Sea

Jason Natural Sea Kelp Shampoo, which smells at bit like a pina colada, contains hair-pampering ingredients such as marigold, chamomile, aloe vera, kukui nut, Hawaiian ginger, plumeria and orchid flowers, amino acids, hydrolyzed chlorophyllin, vitamins E, A, and C, as well as sea kelp. You don't know whether to wash with it or drink it! Jason also has a line of hair conditioners. Their Aloe Vera 84 Conditioner contains vitamins, minerals, spirulina, and 22 keratin amino acids, plus comfrey, marigold, horsetail, jojoba, and vitamins E, D, A and F. It smells fresh and seaworthy.

Especially for Men

Lola Montez advised, "Many a dandy, who has scarcely brains enough or courage enough to catch a sheep, has enslaved the hearts of a hundred girls with his Hyperion locks." When I asked celebrity stylist Gad Cohen how men might improve their looks, he responded: "As mood changes, men should feel free to change their hair, beard, and sideburns. If he normally has a smooth face, let a beard grow for a couple of days. Don't slick back your hair as usual or get a cut." Gad prefers to cut hair during the full moon because he feels it grows back faster and healthier. He recommends regular hair cuts (even for long hair) to help people deal with life's challenges. He says hair is like antennas. It collects information about your life. When you get a cut, it gets rid of outdated material and excess baggage.

Lola's Way

To prevent graying and hair loss, Lola Montez recommended temperance and moderation in all things, as well as frequent washing in pure cold water to cool the head. In *The Arts of Beauty* she wrote, "Perpetual care, great anxiety, or prolonged grief will hasten white hairs. Sudden passion, or grief, or fright have turned head instantly grey."

According to TCM, exhaustion, emotional upset, and chronic illness upset the full range of "kidney" functions (affecting the Water Element), including fertility, sexuality, immunity, and beauty issues. An overheated adrenal output can affect hormone production. That may explain why Lola, not a Chinese doctor but an observer of men and their hair, made the above comment about cooling the head.

Dr. Rudolph Ballentine, in his informative book, *Radical Healing,* suggests hair loss to be from "tightening of scalp due to effort to control the flow of life." He recommends massage and brushing to loosen and relax the scalp. That may follow from the belief that control issues (hyperadrenal) can affect testosterone levels.

Our activity is a soothing scalp massage in a tepid bath. I recommend mixing 3 drops of Australian Tea Tree Oil with 5–10 drops of pure essential oregano oil for the scalp massage. Add Epsom salts to your bath and turn on Bach's "Well Tempered Clavier." The early preludes sound like a relaxed walk. Soak, breathe deeply, gently massage your head with the oil, and visualize taking a long, happy walk.

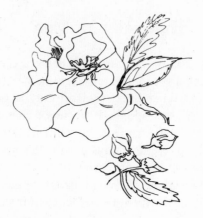

11

Alluring Eyes

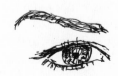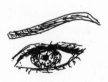

*"The artist must be ready to be consumed by the fire
of his own creation."*
—AUGUSTE RODIN

We begin making love with our eyes. Thinking about the loved one, our gaze softens and turns inward. Our eyes feel moistened as they sink imperceptibly deeper into energy pathways called meridians that link the eyes with the heart and groin. In traditional Chinese medicine, the eyes are part of the Wood Element, which can express the exuberance of spring. Wood controls energetic spheres now considered to be the liver, gall bladder, muscles, tendons, and joints.

The relation of the eyes to the Wood Element is similar to flower petals floating on a lake. If the lake is disturbed by wind or rain, the petals are tossed into the water. If the Wood Element's health is troubled by diet, stress, illness, or upset, the liver cannot produce enzymes necessary to absorb calcium. Then muscles cannot be nourished and circulation suffers. Each part of the energy system reacts on the rest so that eventually we develop eye tics and flutters, pain, or chronic eye problems.

Sexual drive, creative action, and emotional restraint are the dramas played out by the Wood Element's meridians. They pass upward from the big toe along the inner leg to the groin, chest, eyes and brain then downward again from the eyes, neck, shoulders, tops of the arms and hands, down the sides, hips, legs, ankles, and to the fourth toe. This invisible energy loop lets us curl into a ball or spring like a tiger.

Do you have half-shut bedroom eyes or bulging eyes that float in puffy sacs of water retention? How your eyes look is greatly influenced by your lifestyle and beauty products. In this chapter, we will consider both.

The Eyes and the Soul

According to TCM, the Wood Element fuels enthusiasm and carries action to completion. For that reason, the eyes are considered to be the outlet of the "soul." The soul, as explained in the *Nei Jing,* is not a religious concept but an operational function to be observed in diagnosis.

A Chinese doctor notices your posture, movements, and complexion; listens to the quality of your voice; then takes your pulses and looks at your tongue to measure vitality, balance, and immunity to illness. The doctor may search your eyes to check your mental and emotional presence—whether you are able to decide what you want and take rational steps to get it. Can you act from the desires of your "soul," are you scattered and unbalanced by emotions, or are you out to lunch entirely?

Sad or angry people may look away, unable to acknowledge their surroundings. Exhaustion makes puffy, bloodshot eyes sink into pools of water. A wild-eyed fixed glare along with a rapid pulse and deranged speech can signal obsession, madness, or—according to some Asian traditions—demonic possession. Is your circulation quagmired? Does your vitality seem to pour out of your eyes onto a computer screen? Natural treatments that heal and beautify the eyes include herbs and foods that support blood production, circulation, relaxation, and internal moisture. All are deeply rejuvenating.

Things to Avoid

Spicy foods, alcohol, stimulants, overwork, and a sedentary lifestyle all increase acid and irritation throughout the body. If you work late or sleep poorly, your eyes cannot get the rest and nourishment they need. During sleep, our eyes are bathed with moisture. Poor digestion and late meals often result in stomach and chest discomfort or insomnia so that blood circulation to the eyes is reduced. Veins, muscles, and the optic nerve suffer.

Make the Switch from Coffee to Tea

To improve digestion, it is a good idea to switch from coffee to Chinese Pu-Erh (a.k.a. Pu Er tea) and Chrysanthemum flower tea. Pu-Erh, a red tea, is digestive and helps to reduce heartburn. Chrysanthemum flowers ease eye strain and cool the head. Pu Erh and chrysanthemum flowers have been combined in a tea bag found in most shops in Chinatown or online. All Chinese herb and food shops sell big bags of dried yellow chrysanthemum flowers. The tea is best enjoyed between meals. Steep a pinch of the flowers in a glass pot and watch the flowers open as the tea steeps. They are sweet enough to avoid adding sugar. You might also add a handful of dried lycium fruit, another sweet herb famous for eye health and beauty. They relax and refresh the eyes. The tea can be served hot or iced.

Foods and Nutrients for the Eyes

To help clear eye inflammation, increase your vitamin A sources. Eat carrots, asparagus, apricots, musk melon, papaya, peach, prunes, watermelon, and loads of green leafy vegetables. B complex vitamins, especially B1 thiamine (an antistress nutrient), are important. Manganese, found in nasturtium leaves, almonds, black walnuts, watercress, mint, parsley, endive, pineapple, raspberries, apples, avocado, banana, and red currants, is essential for memory, the nervous system, and normal brain functioning. Manganese deficiency symptoms include convulsions, dizziness, facial neuralgia, angry and silent moods, blindness, paralysis, poor muscle coordination, and hearing loss. You may say, "That sounds like old age." But you can help prevent such discomforts with mixed trace minerals including manganese, which is essential for the liver's absorption of calcium.

Recent eye research is focusing on lutein and zeaxanthin, which are abundant in foods such as kale, spinach, fresh parsley, and broccoli. "Lutein and zeaxanthin seem to be most protective in preventing damage to the back of the eye from sunlight and from free radicals (bad guys which can actually kill the cells)," says Dr. Steven Pratt of Scripps Memorial Hospital.

The National Institutes of Health (NIH) is researching whether taking supplements of vitamin C, vitamin E, beta carotene, and zinc can help prevent cataracts and age-related macular degeneration, the leading cause in the United States of irreversible blindness in the elderly. Says Pratt: "Leafy greens may lead the way to eye health." Among greens, I prefer kale, watercress, collards, and chicory as well as various Japanese salad and field greens. I also like adding soaked seaweeds such as arame or hijiki, sources of vitamins and calcium, to salads. Zen Palate, which has three New York locations, makes a nice salad of chopped kale and seaweed with a light sesame vinaigrette dressing.

One traditional Chinese herbal medicine for cataracts is made from equal parts of lycium fruit, rehmannia, astragalus seed, and bat guano (no kidding). To modify this recipe, I cook the first three ingredients in a crockpot set at low heat overnight. With each cup that I drink of the resulting brew, I replace the guano with its vitamin equivalent—10,000 units of vitamin A and 800 units of vitamin D. The result is better-looking, bright eyes and improved vision. The herbal treatment is relaxing for nerves and deeply moistening and rejuvenating for hair, skin, and eyes.

Pills for Enhanced Eye Comfort

All herbal pill formulas for treating eye health and beauty should be used between meals to insure good effects and comfortable digestion.

Caffeine Withdrawal, made by Natra-Bio, is a homeopathic pill remedy that I could recommend in every chapter of this book. Hard work, caffeinated drinks, chocolate, and stress set the jaw, tighten facial muscles, tire and dry out eyes, and make them squint so that you look ready for battle. One or two doses of Caffeine Withdrawal allow your face and eyes to relax without dulling energy and enthusiasm. It contains homeopathic remedies recommended for anger, impatience, upset stomach, nausea, irritability, insomnia, heartburn, and headache. When was the last time you tried to give up coffee but got a headache or the shakes?

Cooling, blood-enhancing Chinese patent formulas such as Mingmu Di Huang Wan (Rehmannia Pills for Improving Eyesight) nourish kidney and liver blood to improve eyesight. The formula contains rehmannia, cornus, moutan bark, dioscurea, poria, alisma, lycium fruit, chrysanthemum flowers, dong quai, tribulus fruit, abalone shell (a source of calcium), and white peony. Moisturizing tonic herbs such as rehmannia and lycium help muscles to relax while they replenish the blood supply to internal organs. Mingmu Di Huang Wan is recommended for blurry vision, watery eyes caused by wind, and night blindness. You can take a handful of pills between meals several times daily. If they are too moistening and laxative, combine them with a digestive tonic such as Xiao Yao Wan.

If you have neck and shoulder tension with blurry vision from overwork, a popular remedy is Head-Q (pills) made by Health Concerns. The formula contains chrysanthemum flowers to cool eyes and reduce blurry vision. Other cooling moistening ingredients include ophiopogon, skullcap, feverfew, and herbs that stimulate circulation such as dong quai and ligusticum.

Healthy Eye Treatment

Shining eyes are beautiful eyes. The following massage advice applies whether or not you currently have eye problems. It can often prevent eye discomforts. As you become involved in creating beauty from top to bottom, you will want to add these treatments to your daily routine.

A Cucumber for Your Eyes

To soothe eyes, apply one of the following onto closed eyes for 10 minutes: a cotton ball dipped into cold fresh milk, a steeped tea bag, or a sliced cucumber.

Eye Massage

Another easy way to reduce eye puffiness is to apply Georgette Klinger's Eye Recovery Gel Mask and then lie down with your feet propped up for 15 minutes. That sends circulation to the head as the eye mask does its magic. It contains firming extracts of witch hazel, cucumber, eyebright herb, cornflower, aloe vera gel, green tea, lecithin, and vitamins E and A in a soothing base that firms and softens lines as it moisturizes the delicate eye area. While the gel mask is working, do the following gentle massage.

Rub the palms of your hands together until warm. Cup them over your closed eyes so that the warmth penetrates. With your fingertips, press under your cheekbones to the front of the ears, along the sides of the neck and tops of the shoulders. Press under your collarbones and down the front of the sternum between the breasts. Pause for a while at the heart and inhale gently. Imagine a pink rose growing there and exhale slowly. Continue smoothing away any sense of tension from the abdomen. Press with both palms on the groin and down the inner thigh and inner knee to the ankles. Turn the ankles around to release tension and wiggle the toes. You will feel relaxed from head to foot.

Lie on your back with your feet elevated for another 10 minutes and then remove the Georgette Klinger Eye Recovery Gel Mask with cotton balls dipped into cool water. If you have sallow or drab skin, tap your face and neck with your fingers to bring more color and blood to your face.

Georgette Klinger's Sea Extracts Eye Cream is a good night cream for puffy eyes and can also be used as a beauty treatment while flying in an airplane because its astringent ingredients (including extracts of sea plankton, bladderwrack seaweed, and algae) reduce puffiness and soothe tired eyes. Avoid using salt and alcohol while flying of if you have missed a night's sleep, because they increase puffy eyes.

Eyebrows Shape the Face

Eyebrows, an essential tool in flirtation, can invite, scold, or announce boredom with the slightest movement. Women have painted, plucked, and tattooed arches from antiquity to today. Clif deRaita, National Director of Makeup at

Georgette Klinger says, "The brows, eyes, and lips are the expression makers, therefore the impression makers." Clif has crafted arches for, among others, Brooke Shields and Senator Hillary Rodham Clinton. He believes that each woman creates an impression and shows her true nature with her eyes: "Brooke Shields' strong eyebrows have always been part of her identity. She is a tall woman. She has strong, beautiful bone structure so that her eyebrows are in perfect balance and she carries that look well." Another hint from Clif: petite women may seem overpowered by their bushy eyebrows.

A Nice Clean Arch for the Fast Track

Does your work show on your brow? Eyebrows not only create facial expression to express mood, but the arch can emphasize the eyes and erase years from the face. Clif deRaita says, "Eyebrows can have a nice clean arch to give the face a lift." For example, Senator Clinton "had a very strong brow," says Clif. He gave her a softer, more elegant expression. I had noticed her new, refined-looking eyebrows once she became a United States senator. They went from bushy to elegant overnight. Clif remarked, "I was the first one to shape her brows. . . . Personalities have to be ready for the camera every minute." Says Clif, "Her look naturally evolved as she has, from a young lawyer to a world traveler who shared the limelight with her famous husband and currently as an influential senator. Her face naturally expresses the change." When I asked him whether Senator Clinton's new eyebrows had anything to do with looking elegant for New Yorkers, he smiled and replied: "Her look expresses her wonderful personality. She is all about beauty that is inside."

A Brow Lift Without Surgery

Do you want a mini-facelift but find yourself short of time and money? Your brows may be the answer. Eliza Petrescu, owner of Eliza's Eyebrow Salon in Avon's Spa and product store in the Trump Tower on Fifth Avenue in New York, believes that inner beauty shows on the face and especially in the brows. Eliza is an eyebrow expert that I predict may start a trend, much like the nail boutiques that mushroomed overnight a few years ago. Her motto is: "Shaping your brows is like getting a seven-minute facelift. Eyebrows balance the face. Unlike the eyes, lips, and nose, the brows are the only thing we can change to look balanced." Eliza says, "Sometimes a person comes with one eyebrow higher or lower. Or the brows are too close or too far apart. I can balance that." She knows that eyebrows indicate emotions. "When you are sad or mad you squint. It changes the eyebrows. I think drooping eyebrows can show a problem with the heart."

Eliza, an Eastern European, easily accepts an aesthetic that comprehends beauty inside and out. She feels that any client of hers will have mind, body, emotions, habits, and eyebrows that should work together for a look of balance and harmony. Eyebrows might also signify emotional problems that don't exist. The heroin-chic, black-eyed look of starvation currently popular with some designers is one example. When *Vogue* magazine interviewed Eliza about it for their July 2001 issue, she said: "Life is not a stage. Trends come and go. It's better to have a natural look."

Pencil-Thin Brows or No Brows

A few women tweeze their brows almost completely off and draw in a thin pencil line to make a fake brow, resembling Jean Harlow or Betty Boop. Eliza thinks they are nervous or scared. Gad Cohen, a famous New York stylist whom I have quoted throughout the book, says, "Pencil-thin eyebrows are an old lady look." He prefers smoothing brows in their natural direction with a powder and brush. He often uses a slightly darker or contrasting color to give a soft, natural look.

Eye adornment styles may change as fashion dictates, but a deeper issue is always involved. Lyn is a very attractive Connecticut-based psychotherapist who helps people with food and substance abuse and depression, which she calls denial of life and the body. "It's the unhealthy ways of coping with stress that we suffer from most." She seems very well balanced emotionally and obviously takes good care of herself with regular beauty treatments.

Trichotillomania is the jaw-breaker term used by her profession to describe the neurosis of plucking out one's own eyebrows and hair. "People who pluck to extreme then draw pencil-thin eyebrows do not trust what is natural and real about themselves. Usually they are put on antidepressant drugs," she said. To a therapist, heroin chic is not a fashion statement but indicates that the person does not feel alive. As Lyn says, "They do not trust their beauty."

Lyn continued: "What's beautiful is someone running on the beach with the wind in their face, laughing with friends, playing with their pet—its health and acceptance of life and vitality. A depressed person, alcoholic, or addict *cannot* look you in the eye when they speak. It's too painful. They look all around. They are not present. I have my patients look at themselves in the mirror daily and say, 'I love you just the way you are.' That is the beginning of accepting the body, life, and being real."

Your Perfect Eyebrows

If you are not quite ready to accept yourself yet, here is expert beauty advice on how to shape the perfect brow. It's easy.

- Trim your brows. Use a round brow brush or clean mascara wand to sweep brow hair up above the brow line, then trim any long hairs with tiny brow scissors. Brush brow hairs down and repeat, trimming hairs that fall below the arch.
- Locate the inner brow edge. Use a brow pencil or straight nail file. Lay the pencil vertically along the right side of your nose. Where it hits your brow is where the inside starting point of your right brow should be. Mark that point on the right and repeat for the left brow in the same way. Remove hairs that fall between those points.
- Locate the outer brow edge. Hold the bottom of the pencil at the center of your bottom lip, letting the top of the pencil slant out to the outside edge of your right eye. Where the inside edge of the pencil hits is where your brow should end. Mark this spot with the pencil and do the same on the left side.
- Find the high point of the arch. Hold the base of the pencil at the center of your bottom lip and slant it out until the inside edge lies just along the outside edge of your iris (the colored part of your eye). The highest point of the arch should be where the inside edge of the pencil meets your eyebrow.
- Sketch in the shape of the brow with an eyebrow pencil. Tweeze or wax hairs that do not conform with the shape. Sterilize the tweezer with rubbing alcohol before using it. Pull hair out in the direction of the hair growth.
- Lightly powder the brow with the appropriate color. Eyebrow powder gives a softer finish than paint or pencil.
- Lift your eyes, brows, and forehead by braiding your hair or pulling it back off your face. Then attach a hairpiece pony tail or a heavy hair clip to make the facial skin taut.

For Younger Eyes

When your body is completely relaxed, you feel as though the tiny bones in your hands and feet have more space between them; that your spine, legs, and arms are longer and more graceful; and that your eyes have adequate moisture reaching them from the deep recesses that contain their blood supply. This exercise will bring a shine to your eyes and reduce the puffiness underneath.

Apply your favorite eye mask such as Georgette Klinger's Eye Mask Gel or light, creamy, and nourishing Virtual Perfection Eye Care, which contains avocado oil, jewelweed extract, wheat protein, and willow bark extract. Use a circular motion beginning upward at the inside corners and across the top near the eyebrow, then tap lightly with fingertips at the outside corners.

Lie on a slant or flat in a quiet space placing a tube pillow beneath your neck and under the backs of your knees to support them. Place your hands on top of your thighs or at your sides. Take one dose of homeopathic ruta grav. 30C every 15 minutes for up to an hour. Close your eyes and imagine the space inside your eyes to be perfectly black. After resting, remove the eye mask with warm water and spray your face with rose water to balance your skin's pH.

A Quick Fix Tea for Computer Eyes

Are your eyes glued to the screen? *Prunella vulgaris* tea (also called self-heal or heal-all, and in Chinese xia ku cao) promotes healing for irritated computer eyes because it relaxes the area all around the eyes as it reduces swelling and eye dryness. Sometimes combined with other herbs for goiters or neck and breast lumps, it works specifically to relax and refresh the liver meridian as it passes through the eyes. It helps to reduce the bulging-eye look of a hyper-thyroid condition.

Brew a handful of the dried herb in your teapot and drink it warm or cool without honey. If you have irritated eyes, insomnia, facial blemishes, or nervousness, add one tube of Chinese pearl powder to steep with the tea. It makes a nice drink before bed especially if bad dreams make you squirm and squint.

Especially for Men

Why let women be the only ones with attractive eyes? Bloodshot eyes make you look as though you have not slept. They signal stress, worry, fatigue, and other uncool things that might interfere with an "I can do anything" impression. Keep some natural eye drops that contain pearl in your drawer at work. If you are nervous and hyper, drink prunella tea plain or sweetened with Essence of Tienchi Flowers Chinese instant beverage as needed. For puffy eyes from overindulgence or lack of sleep, pour hot water over two caffeine tea bags, squeeze them to damp, and apply them to closed eyes for 15 minutes instead of taking a cigarette break.

Thick brows were fine for Captain Ahab in *Moby Dick*, but there is no advantage in hiding your eyes under rugs. You will see better if you trim them. One of my actor friends was nervous about an interview with one of Broadway's top directors. He got his hair color touched up and his long lashes permed, which made his eyes look bigger and bluer. The beauty expert smiled, "Honey, don't show your mother, but you look great!" My friend got the job, which paid enormously. Taking care of business means always taking care of your looks.

Lola's Way

A car can't go far without headlights. Your spirit expresses itself in your actions, words, and thoughts, as well as your vision of who you are in relation to others. Sick or neurotic people become short-sighted in their desires and range of emotions as their vision of the future shrinks. Hatred is one of the most dangerous emotions because, like desire itself, it can never be satisfied. Fear constricts our movements and desires for future happiness.

Dr. Rudolph Ballentine, a delightfully mystical New York medical doctor, writes in *Radical Healing,* "Cataracts is not wanting to see the future—especially elderly who have materialistic concepts of death." He recommends local irritants such as cineraria eye drops, yellow mustard oil, or lotus honey—a drop in each eye twice daily. Dr. Christopher's herbal eye wash is made with powdered bayberry bark, euphrasia, raspberry, and goldenseal in equal parts with 1/8 as much cayenne powder. Steep 1 teaspoon of the powder in one cup of boiling distilled water, decant, cool, and use it in a glass eye cup two to five times daily to bring mucus discharge.

East Indian herbalists link cataracts with hypertension and poor circulation. Most Western scientists believe the lens becomes dry from excess sun exposure at high altitudes. Many children in Nepal get cataracts. Whatever the cause of dryness—emotional unrest, poor blood circulation, sun, or chemical exposure—you can moisten eyes and reduce eyestrain daily with soothing Pearl Drops from Chinatown (or from internet sources for Chinese herbs listed at the back of this book).

Pearl represents a recurrent theme in this book on natural beauty. Used internally, as Chinese Pearl Powder added to water, its minerals add luster to eyes and complexion. Pearl reduces redness and irritation from the skin, hypertension, infantile fever and convulsions, as well as menopausal hot flashes—pearl nurtures beauty at all ages. Pearls, the gem and the medicine, epitomize the link between internal vitality and healthy beauty. The following three chapters address a flawless complexion, which arises from harmony within.

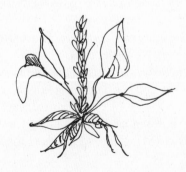

12

Your Flawless Complexion

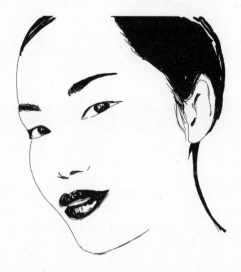

"Though it is true that a beautiful mind is the first
thing requisite for a beautiful face, yet how much
more charming will the whole become through the aid
of a fine complexion?"
—LOLA MONTEZ

Our outer envelope, linked to pathways of breathing and elimination, is our most superficial organ. Many people spend a fortune on blemish or wrinkle treatments or pass hours self-scrutinizing in front of a mirror. In traditional Chinese medicine, skin is an extension of our lungs and large intestine, which make up the Metal Element, an organ system within which we hold breath and emotions. Ancient Chinese doctors felt that each Element housed a spirit (*shen*) to maintain its emotional well-being. The lungs are said to contain *Po,* the spirit necessary for self-preservation. People with a tendency towards shallow breathing, mucus congestion, and chronic blemishes were thought to suffer more acutely from sadness. A healthy *Po* offered protection against habits such as smoking and drugs. Our fascination in front of a mirror may be our attempt to visually comprehend our emotions.

Breathing is a survival issue for all who live in cities. Smoking and breathing polluted air lead to a thick, rough, sallow, and gray complexion. Clear, glowing skin is possible only when blood and cells are bathed in oxygen. You can greatly improve your vitality and mood by addressing complexion because its beauty is founded on digestion and respiration, which eliminate toxins. Many cleansing herbs and foods used to prevent and treat blemishes increase all sorts of deep-cleansing. As congestion and impurities are dislodged, you may feel physically and emotionally unburdened. The best way to achieve beautiful skin is by eliminating impurities and stress, which weaken all internal organs.

Skin-Tech

According to Lola Montez, "the great secret of acquiring a bright and beautiful skin lies in three simple things—temperance, exercise, and cleanliness." Her "villains" described in *The Arts of Beauty* were a breakfast of strong coffee, hot bread, and butter. "Hot grease is sure to derange the stomach, and by creating or increasing bilious disorders, gradually overspreads the fair skin with a wan or yellow hue." In her lectures on beautiful women, Lola warns against fasting all day then eating a rich spicy dinner (including peppered soups; fish; roast, boiled, broiled, and fried meat or game; and tarts, sweet meats, ices, and fruits). The inevitable result she says is: "The heated complexion bears witness to the combustion within!"

People have done horrific things to themselves in quest of complexion beauty. Lola reported that Bohemian girls drank from arsenic-rich springs and soon after died. Women from the court of George I took minute doses of quicksilver (mercury) and became ill. It is true that homeopathic arsenicum has been used for herpes simplex and mercurius for boils. However, correct homeopathic preparation and dosage are essential. Since Lola's day, homeopathic use of dangerous substances has been standardized.

During the 1850s girls ate chalk, slate, and tea grounds for a fair complexion. The latter at least sounds closer to an herbal answer. Tea is cleansing and very beneficial for the entire body because of its powerful antioxidants and catechins, which are concentrated acids with anticholesterol properties.

Lola's suggestion for a radiant complexion was, "frequent ablution with pure cold water, followed by gentle and very frequent rubbing with a dry napkin." Exfoliants have come a long way since her time. Nevertheless, many remain unsafe. One popular acne drug is so drying when swallowed that it reportedly increases sexual discomfort and panic. That means it increases blood acidity, which may lead to dangerous consequences. Natural beauty remedies take longer to work than drugs, but they are proven safe and effective over time.

The Face in the Mirror

Daily habits show up on the skin because complexion is affected by factors deeper than climate, germs, and pollution. Your face is a map of your energy, digestion, and elimination. Facial redness, irritation, and acne can improve fast with a simple cleansing diet made up of 60% raw foods, which supply oxygen. It includes white rice, steamed or baked fish, fresh vegetables, raw and steamed red cabbage, cooling cucumber, fruits, seaweeds, nuts, raw seeds, and 5–10 cups daily of green tea.

An excellent skin-beautifying tea is alfalfa, dandelion, and peppermint made using dried herbs or pills. Empty 3 capsules of each powdered herb into a porcelain teapot and steep in boiling water for 10 minutes before drinking three to five cups daily. Alfalfa is full of necessary minerals. Dandelion cleanses the skin and especially the blood of impurities. Peppermint is digestive and soothing. Dr. Bernard Jensen's oatstraw and black cherry tea that I recommended in Chapter 10 for the hair is also beneficial for complexion.

The best raw juices for complexion are fresh parsley, cucumber, carrot, endive, apple, and pineapple. You might juice the fruits in the morning and the vegetables in the afternoon for a quick energy and beauty lift. Fruits by nature are more acidic than vegetables. You will want to feel more cool as the day goes on. Otherwise, acidic fruits eaten at night might lead to nervous hunger. Parsley, cucumber, and endive are bitter cleansers that eliminate acid impurities. Carrot is rich in beneficial vitamins such as C and A. Apple and pineapple work to reduce mucus congestion throughout the body. Skin blemishes remain intractable when excess mucus clogs elimination.

An delicate tea from China called Cherry Grain Balsam Pear Tea is available in some Chinese supermarkets and online. It comes in a box showing the Yangtze Basin's beautiful tapestry of green and yellow fields and blue skies in China's Jiangsu Province. The tea inside is no less spectacular. Described by some as "clear and elegant" in flavor, it contains no tea (camellia sinensis) or caffeine but dried slices of a bitter gourd that is known by a dozen names such as bitter melon, towel gourd, tiansigua, tianluo, and xugua. People who complain about tea's "muddy" taste often love this beverage served hot or cold. For a mild tea, steep two or three pieces of dried bitter melon tea (Balsam Pear Tea) in a cup of hot water. I also add a handful of the dried slices to soups or recipes for a tart flavor.

The tea is a popular daily remedy throughout Asia and the Caribbean for cooling and cleansing the body from fever, thirst, agitation, diabetes, cough, and phlegm congestion anywhere—for the nose and throat or for vaginal discharge. Balsam Pear Tea especially acts on the liver and stomach meridians to "cool and cleanse the blood." That means its components, including saponins and vitamins B and C, reduce impurities that might lead to inflammatory problems such as bad breath, thirst, or a bloody nose.

Usually when a friend asks for tea in my home, I look at their tongue the way any traditional Chinese doctor would to diagnose what they might need. I serve a cup of Cherry Grain Balsam Pear Tea if the tongue is dry, reddish, or coated with yellow mucus. I also give it to anyone with PMS, hot flashes, irritability, complexion blemishes, or excess weight, as well as anyone who smokes, eats too many hot spices, or frequently drinks alcohol. That covers just about everyone. If you still have complexion problems after changing your diet, the specific guide that follows will help you. Notice blemishes on corresponding areas of the face. Watch problems clear as you add the suggested foods and herbs to your diet.

- The forehead corresponds to the intestines. For blemishes, eat laxative yellow vegetables such as squash, pumpkin, and carrot, which are high in vitamin A. For horizonal lines and dryness from dehydration or chronic diarrhea, replenish mixed trace minerals and especially vitamin B15 (a.k.a. DMG or pure N,N-dimethylglycine).
- Squint-lines between the eyes corresponds to stress, blood deficiency, and a hyperactive liver. Cleanse and build your liver with lots of green vegetables—high in chlorophyll and oxygen—especially watercress. Anti-stress supplements include 60–100 mg daily of zinc. A daily dose of cod liver oil taken along with evening primrose oil will nourish the liver.
- Cheeks correspond to stomach, spleen, and pancreas. A wan or pasty complexion shows poor absorption of nutrients. Blemishes and fragile capillaries show excess acids and blood poverty. Daily herbs that reduce digestive acid include aloe vera, peppermint, alfalfa, and dandelion. Licorice tea is also said to be soothing for ulcers and excess acid.
- Your chin shows reproductive organs and hormone balance. Breakouts can indicate a difficult period. Sarsaparilla tea is effective for hormone- or stress-related acne. Gotu kola herb and tea are useful for calming anxiety-related blemishes.

Special Complexion Beauty Problems

Acne

Stubborn, deep pimples do not always improve with washing. Scrubbing increases oily skin. Excess oil and impurities must be addressed at their source with internal cleansing. Among traditional Chinese herbs there are everyday teas and pills that can be used for acne prevention and treatment. The following Chinese herbal formulas for acne contain antibiotic and antiinflammatory cleansing herbs used for regulating the blood and intestines while reducing acids and impurities. They treat itching and skin inflammation for conditions ranging from acne, psoriasis, eczema, rosacea, and hives. If an outbreak occurs while you are working on unrelated issues, step up your dosage of cleansing/laxative herbs such as those that follow.

A Liver Cleansing Tea

Yin/Yang Sisters instant beverages will be discussed in detail in later chapters concerning toxic pollution, germ warfare, and rejuvenation remedies. Among the eight varieties currently available, Clean Habits, a powerful herbal liver and blood cleaner, is most appropriate for eliminating stubborn acne, carbuncles, eczema, and boils. Empty the contents of one foil-wrapped package into a cup and add hot water. Drink the beverage hot or cold one to three times daily as needed. It can be sweetened with a complexion-beautifying Chinese sugar substitute such as Sheshecao Beverage crystals.

Chinese Herbal Pills

Lien Chiao Pai Tu Pien, a Chinese herbal pill, is made up of antifever, antibiotic, and laxative herbs such as honeysuckle flower, forsythia, and rhubarb. The dosage is 4 pills taken twice daily. For stronger action, they can be taken along with capsules of *Oldenlandia diffusa* (bai hua sheshecao) for carbuncles, boils, and stubborn acne. Chinese antibiotic herbs such as this have been used with confidence for generations. While using them, take acidophilus or yogurt adding a pinch of turmeric powder to rebalance your digestive flora.

Skin Balance, made by Health Concerns, are pills that contain skullcap, oldenlandia, gentian, rehmannia, viola, siler, lonicera, lysimachia, coptis root, tang kuei, bupleurum, carthamus, senna leaf, and rhubarb. They are recommended to reduce itching and skin inflammation, and remove toxins in the blood that lead to inflammation as they moisten and nourish complexion. I like to explain herbal combinations such as this one because they are wisely put together. The herbs work well together to help clear liver inflammation and impurities by stimulating cleansing.

Viola, lonicera, and oldenlandia are plants that have antibiotic properties. Skullcap and coptis are cooling and cleansing for the liver and digestive tract. They also move impurities from the blood. Rehmannia and tang kuei insure proper blood production and circulation. Rhubarb, lysimachia, senna, and carthamus remove wastes because they are laxative. The standard dosage for Skin Balance is 3 tablets three or four times daily. Reduce dosage if diarrhea occurs.

Such herbal combinations work by speeding the body's natural methods of purification. It seems obvious, however you have to look closer to understand. Skin impurities require bitter, sour, and pungent laxative and diuretic herbs—not sweet or hot diaphoretic herbs and foods. Even healthy sweets such as orange juice and honey, because they are diaphoretic (encourage sweating), bring excess acid to the skin. Skin eruptions increase by using sweat-inducing foods or natural sweating from exercise and stress.

Trifala Churna, the All-in-One Cleanser Healer

Trifala Churna, a powerfully rejuvenating herbal powder available in all East Indian groceries, contains three rejuvenating fruits suitable for people of all ages. They are amla (*Emblica officinalis*), bibhitaki (*Terminalia belerica*), and haritake (*Terminalia chebula*). Trifala powder (churna) is a popular cleanser/ balancer for a multitude of health and beauty issues. Used daily, it tones and rejuvenates the skin, lungs, liver, and colon. As a gentle cleanser/rejuvenator, you can add ¼ teaspoon of Trifala powder to hot water as a tea, fill an empty capsule with the powder, or drink a cup of "Get Regular" Yogi Tea from the supermarket twice daily.

Amla is one of the highest known sources of vitamin C, with 3000 mg per fruit. It cleanses the mouth and strengthens teeth and gums, nourishes the bones, and causes hair and nails to grow. It improves eyesight and reduces stomach and colon inflammation.

Bibhitake is a tonic to the lungs and improves the voice. It is recommended for cough, sore throat, laryngitis, bronchitis, chronic diarrhea, and parasites. Haritake, sometimes called one of the most important Ayurvedic herbs, feeds the brain and nerves. It is also recommended for cough, asthma, malabsorption, abdominal distention and parasites, tumors, jaundice, heart disease, skin diseases, itching, edema, and nervous disorders. (In Chinese, it is called he zi.) The herb does so many things, especially reduce dis-ease, that in Sanskrit it is called *abhaya*—it promotes fearlessness. The combination of these three fruits in Trifala Churna make it a supreme cleansing and balancing remedy. I recommend 1/4 teaspoon in hot water as a tea twice daily.

Dark Circles

Dark circles under the eyes often result from fatigue and allergies. One fine remedy for both is nettle tea. Once a friend sat in my apartment suffering from her cat-fur allergy. I gave her a cup of hot nettle tea and she was amazed—no more choking, tearing, and coughing. Eventually, her allergies and dark circles were eliminated by drinking an afternoon pot of nettle tea along with her daily zinc supplement.

Dull, Lifeless Skin

A high-stress lifestyle requires adequate oxygen in the cells. I add doses of homeopathic potassium and iron to my morning pot of green tea. Per pot add 5 pills each of homeopathic kali mur. (potassium chloride); kali sulph. (potassium sulphate); and ferrum phosphate (iron) all at 6x strength. Drink this tea one hour before or after meals. Soon your skin will breathe again.

Eczema

Dandelion and honeysuckle flower tea is especially useful for chronic itchy rashes and eczema. Simmer a handful of each herb in 1 quart of water for 20 minutes and drink one to three cups daily. This laxative brew is gentle enough for children and animals when used in doses of no more than one cup daily. The best homeopathic remedy for eczema is homeopathic sulphur 30C. It especially addresses redness and itching. You need to use it three to five times daily for at least one month and avoid sugar, coffee, and alcohol. The homeopathic remedy may help you to avoid these temptations.

Bug Bites

For the last several years, West Nile virus has been carried by mosquitoes. Central Park was sprayed with insecticide and New Yorkers were warned by health authorities to stay indoors whenever possible. Yeah, right! We have enough to worry about in New York without mosquitoes. Aside from being health hazards, bug bites mar complexion. New Englanders are expert about insect repellents. Some amusing, home-tested solutions date from the Civil War. One is to drink a mixture of one cup of apple cider vinegar to a gallon of water. Bugs are attracted to sweet, acidic body odor and vinegar purifies the body. Bugs don't appreciate the smell of garlic either—but then few of us do. B complex vitamins and zinc supplements also detract mosquitoes.

My favorite DEET-free repellent is Natrapel made by Tender Corporation in Littleton, New Hampshire (www.tendercorp.com). It contains only citronella (which smells vaguely lemony), water, aloe vera, vanillin, lauryl sulfate, xanthan gum, potassium sorbate, and citric acid. It is the best, lightest, most pleasant-to-wear repellant that I have found. Usually, they are a gooey, smelly, sticky mess. This one is nice enough to wear alone during day or evening.

Bumps and Warts

One amusing herbal epiphany for skin came to me in the form of a homeopathic thuja ointment made by Washington Homeopathic Products. It is not appropriate for everyone. Thuja Ointment contains homeopathic thuja occ. 1x strength in a base that is half lanolin and petroleum. Used internally or externally, homeopathic thuja is recommended for removing hard, crusty growths, especially warts, corns, and calluses. In the process, it brings them out to the surface of the skin. (There's the rub!)

I applied the cream as a thick, gooey face cream to deep cleanse. I told my friends that I was preventing bunions on my face. After about one week to one month of nightly use, you get an outcrop of warts, blemishes, or bumps that last for a week or more—and then completely fall off. For a while, you feel as though you are dredging up everything and letting it all hang out. You have to step up cleansing by adding herbal pills such as those I recommended in this chapter. Be very careful when applying exfoliants or irritants near fragile or red facial capillaries. Irritants may look and feel red hot and may further damage the skin or increase rosacea.

Rosacea

Rosacea (red or purple broken capillaries, roughness and redness, sometimes with tiny blemishes or bumps on the face) seems to affect blonde, blue-eyed women over 40 more than anyone. Their skin is transparent compared to those with thicker skin and darker complexions. Some doctors also believe that hormonal factors are indirectly involved. Chinese doctors describe as "internal heat" or "false fire" those conditions that resemble inflammation.

The first thing to do is to reduce your intake of hot and spicy foods, caffeine, and alcohol, all of which are inflammatory. One beauty specialist especially recommends eating red cabbage to "bring inflammation away from the face towards the stomach and intestines to be eliminated." Here is a recipe you can enjoy daily.

Steamed or Raw Red Cabbage

Ingredients:
1 red cabbage
1 raw carrot
¼ cup dried raisins
¼ cup pecans
¼ tsp cumin powder
¼ tsp fennel powder
1 Tbsp walnut or grapeseed oil
¼ tsp vanilla extract

1 package of Sheshecao Instant Beverage
1 tube of Chinese pearl powder (optional)

Cut half of the cabbage into large pieces and blanch them for a moment under hot water. Rinse off the raisins and nuts. Blend all ingredients together in a blender until the cabbage is in small slices. At this point you can add a tablespoon of water along with the tube of pearl powder and lightly steam the cabbage or serve the dish raw.

Rosacea is considered by some to be a form of acne. It sometimes looks and feels as though heartburn is rising to spread to the neck and face, leaving permanent redness, tiny bumps, and broken capillaries.The normal Western medical treatment is a lifelong dose of daily antibiotics, which risks ruining digestion and eventually energy and blood production.

As a beautifying treatment for inflamed skin and nervous conditions, many Chinese people swallow 1 or 2 capsules of powdered sea pearl daily. Pearl powder, high in calcium carbonate, clears the complexion as it quiets the nerves. I stir it into cooked oatmeal to cool my skin and nerves. Give your-self a beauty gift. Wing Hop Fung, Los Angeles' largest store selling Chinese ginseng and China products, has a beauty kit that contains pure pearl powder, pearl cream, and several cooling, cleansing instant beverages, including the Sheshecao Instant Beverage (mentioned above). You can order it directly from their website at www.winghopfung.com.

One New York plastic surgeon that I asked about rosacea recommended a gentle massage of the affected area in order to increase circulation. I prefer spreading a homeopathic arnica montana 30C cream or ointment on to the skin instead of applying any pressure. Arnica montana reduces bruising, swelling, and inflammation by naturally increasing circulation.

Other cooling skin creams include 999 Cream, a camphorated white cream in a tube made by 999, one of China's largest herb manufacturers. Any lotion that contains Ester C will also cool complexion. Ester C is the newly discovered antiinflammatory form of vitamin C. It works very well to boost immunity and beauty without the usual acid burn to the stomach. It has been shown to reduce skin redness when used regularly. In your health-food store, see Jason Cosmetics and Kiss My Face for especially fine, all-natural skin products.

A Quick Fix for New Skin

For people on the go, a good way to properly wash and exfoliate the skin is with cleansing grains. Sometimes you can get a combination that includes natural ingredients and an irritant exfoliant. One made by Pro-Beauty Treatments is Soothing Gel Mask, which contains algae extract, vitamin C, glycolic acid, aloe, lemon grass extract, and cucumber. It has a natural, light, grainy feel. Massage for about a minute and leave it on for 10.

For dry, puffy, or aging skin, Kiss My Face Chinese Botanical Moisturizer combines nourishing Chinese asparagus and jujube red date, cooling chrysanthemum, healing kudzu and peonia roots, antioxidant and moistening mulberry twig, as well as diuretic fuling and schisandra (wu wei zi) to help tone facial muscles and reduce excess water retention.

Bird's Nest for Skin Like Silk

Lan Ong, part-owner of Wing Hop Fung, Los Angeles Chinatown's superstore, is soft-spoken and gracefully slender with long, jet hair and enchanting eyes. Lan has the eternal allure that draws us to the East. Her complexion is flawless white with pores made invisible from drinking bird's nest extract. To prepare bird's nest using the traditional recipe, it has to be soaked, cleaned, then steamed in a crockpot for several hours. Lucky for us, it is sold ready-made in cans. For complexion perfection, drink one can of Bird's Nest Extract made with American ginseng and rock sugar daily between meals. It refreshes, reduces thirst, and helps prevent blemishes and wrinkles. Avoid it during a cold or flu.

Especially for Men

Treat yourself or that special guy to a facial, face or body waxing treatment, massage, slimming body wrap, invigorating body rub, or manicure or pedicure at Nickel, New York's exclusive men-only spa imported from Paris. For now, its only U.S. location is in chic Chelsea, but I predict Nickel will spread across America as it did in Europe. Thirty-eight-year-old founder, Philippe Dumont, who has worked with Chanel and Christian Dior, started Nickel (slang for spotless) in a large converted marble bank at the corner of 14th Street and Eighth Avenue. The spa, complete with trickling water and soothing lights, plush robes and comfy slippers, is not open to female perusal.

Nickel products have cool blue and metallic silver packaging and containers that resemble motor oil cans, heavy duty detergents or gasoline cans, and wine bottles. They have a clean soap and spice fragrance and some unique food ingredients. Nickel Super Clean scrubbing gel has pistachio extract for enhanced skin elasticity.

The French love coffee so much that Nickel uses caffeine in several products to boost circulation and tone tired skin. Lendemain de fete ("the day after the party") combines green coffee extract, menthol, witch hazel, and soy proteins as a shock treatment. It gives tired, puffy skin a rush (not recommended for rosacea).

Amuse Gueule (something to amuse your face as well as slang for a toy or trinket) is a deep-acting moisturizer in little blue plastic ampules. Their brochure reads, "Whether you've been hiking all day, clubbing 'til dawn, traveling trans-Atlantic, a few drops of this potion instantly uplifts and softens skin. . . . Simply toss the single-dosage container into your Gucci carry-on or conceal one in your suit pocket for an unexpected night of unconditional passion." They can't help it—they're French. Nickel Massage Canaille oil contains hot pepper to put more spice into your life.

A Close Shave Without Ouch

I asked my men friends about their favorite natural shave cream, and they said that Tom's of Maine makes a cooling, minty cream that contains coconut and olive oils and glycerin. This non-soap cream washes off squeaky clean. For dry or blemished skin, several recommended Jason's Witch Vera as an aftershave. It is made from 84% aloe gel and contains cooling witch hazel, marigold, chamomile, comfrey, and chlorophyll.

The closest shave was reported for Blade Runner by Origins. It conditions the skin with kukui nut oil (*Aleurites molucanna*), sunflower oil, and soy oil and contains a list of energizing herbs, including rosemary, mint, sage, lavender, sandalwood, eucalyptus, geranium, coriander, and kelp. For good measure, it also contains a dash of caffeine to wake up your face every morning. Follow it with Origins' Fire Fighter to take the burn out of shaving. Its chamomile, cucumber, eucalyptus, mint, oats, green tea, and aloe protect skin softness. The Origins shave cream and aftershave give a baby's skin finish.

Lola's Way

Bioplasma is the name given to a combination of 12 homeopathic mineral salts (a.k.a. Schuessler's biochemic tissue remedies or cell salts). Each dose contains minerals essential for cell nourishment and oxygen absorption. Lacking these essential minerals, the skin's cellular activity cannot continue.They assure growth, health, and beauty. Twice daily between meals you should take one dose of Bioplasma (5 pills) in a little water along with 4 pills of a cleansing complexion remedy such as Lien Chiao Pai Tu Pien or Skin Balance.

Sit quietly alone where you will not be disturbed for 30 minutes to an hour. Breathe slowly from the lower abdomen and imagine a beautiful garden growing inside. You can protect and nurture your garden this way anytime you like. Visualize each tree and flower. Consider how well you care for them. Your inner garden is your source of energy and inspiration.

The following two chapters describe topical products and methods to prevent and treat skin imperfections and makeup to enhance your natural gifts.

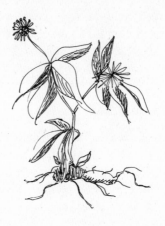

13

Out, Out Damned Spots

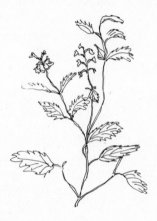

"Oh, would that I could live up to my blue china!"
—OSCAR WILDE

You may have an impressive collection of hats and scarves; cover your face with sunscreen, insect repellant, and thick pancake makeup; or avoid the sun completely. Chances are you still have sunspots, moles, freckles, birthmarks, or other spots.

I had a lifelong problem with spots until writing this chapter. For me, they were part of being Hungarian, along with a taste for spicy foods and romantic music. Bela Lugosi's vampire smile reveals a dark mole on his cheek. Some say moles come from temperament. Tibetans believe that moles are karmic—properly analyzed by an astrologer, they reveal past lives and future potential. My Tibetan astrological chart predicts I will become either an artist or a religious mystic in my next life because I have a mole on my left buttock. I refuse to remove it for that reason.

Chinese herbalists believe moles reflect the health of blood circulation and the liver. The liver's energy (qi) is said to be disturbed by anger. Rage is common for Hungarians. Director Michael Curtiz, known for movie classics including *Casablanca,* never lost his thick accent. While shooting the famous ending, where Elsa and her dissident husband are about to escape by plane, Curtiz shouted, "Poodles, I want poodles!" Confused, his assistants scoured the area for dogs. But Curtiz wanted rain *puddles* on the flying field. Jumping up and down, the director yelled, "Do as I think, not as I say!"

A traditional Chinese herbalist is part mystic, artist, and scientific observer. Like Hahnemann, the eighteenth-century father of homeopathy, I have often used myself and friends as subjects. My experimentation tends to be more audacious than most recommended treatments because I can remedy side effects. Sometimes the results are spectacular. This summer, I attacked spots that mar complexion. With Hussar courage, I tried numerous methods, leaving some in the dust. Now I am nearly spotless.

Moles and Spots

Everyone has skin spots, moles, freckles, birthmarks, or age spots that are harmless. We are born with them, and they come and go. Determining their origin is an interesting problem. The Western medical consensus is that moles and spots, which are made of thicker pigmentation than the surrounding skin, should be checked regularly and treated medically because they increase the risk of skin cancer. You can't even get general information about spots without hearing about skin cancer. A sudden or marked change in moles can mean trouble that requires immediate intervention. Doctors believe that long exposure to the sun should be avoided at all costs. Other contributing factors may include a nutritional deficiency of vitamin C, vitamin E, and beta carotene and age.

Visit a beauty salon in an Asian community and you will hear a different story. Beauty shop owners in New York's Chinatown say moles are a matter of diet and poor circulation. I was warned to avoid shellfish, soy sauce, red meat, hot spices, coffee, and black tea. Many Chinese salons remove small moles without fuss with an electric needle for a minimal price. They cater to Chinese women, who on the whole are familiar with Chinese herbs used for a wide number of health/beauty issues from menopausal hot flashes to skin changes and hair loss. Chinese blood-enhancing herbs assure internal moisture that maintains youth and beauty.

I gladly frequent popular Chinese, Japanese, and Vietnamese salons in New York and Los Angeles that specialize in various forms of dermabrasion and spot removal. Several new Bloomies, specializing in facials and diamond dermabrasion, have moved into my Chelsea neighborhood. Their Asian staff is friendly, and they offer a package deal at a reduced rate. On Madison Avenue, I go to elegant Georgette Klinger for expert individualized treatments including non-irritating dermabrasion.

You can have problematic moles checked for warning signals at clinics such as the New York Hospital dermatology clinic, which is part of Charles C. Harris Skin and Cancer Unit at New York University Medical Center, located at 30th Street and First Avenue. Doctors there are used to looking at moles, spots, and freckles all day. They can remove and analyze the usual suspects on the spot.

Troubleshooting for Moles or Spots

It is important to notice sudden or extreme changes in skin spots. According to www.webMD.com, things doctors look for when trouble shooting are moles that are larger than a pencil eraser; asymmetrical; irregularly shaped; or contain shades of red, blue, white, or black. Another potential problem is skin tags (small skin "stalks" or flap-like growths, usually on the neck, armpits, upper trunk, and body folds) that become red, inflamed, or painful. Finally, yellow, brown, or black growths on the face, chest, shoulders, and back that are slightly raised, waxy, or gritty, and may be more than an inch in diameter, should be checked.

Consult your doctor immediately if any spot or mole suddenly changes in size, height, shape, or color; or if it bleeds, itches, or becomes painful, or infected. Elizabeth Smoots, MD, FAAFP, is a board-certified family physician in Seattle who specializes in prevention and primary care medicine. In a November 20, 2000, article on www.webMD.com she describes these "ABCs" for observing moles:

- A is for asymmetry. If you divide the mole in half, the two parts do not match. Asymmetry may be a sign of cancer.
- B is for border. Irregular edges that are ragged or notched may be a suspicious sign.
- C is for color. Uneven or multiple colors that may vary from brown, black, and pink to red, white, and blue can signal melanoma, a type of skin cancer that can be deadly.
- D is for diameter. A mole may be abnormal if it is bigger than a pencil eraser.
- E is for elevation. A raised or uneven mole can be a sign of skin cancer.

High-Risk Factors

I am considered at high risk for skin cancer because I am blonde, female, and Caucasian. Another factor is that I was exposed to bright sunshine in New Mexico from the ages of 6 to 20. However, other factors balance the scales. One major consideration is that I do not smoke.

The sun has been with us a long time, but pollution has greatly increased over the years. Deforestation and rampant use of chemicals and pesticides have endangered earth's air, water, soil, and ecological balance. Many health experts believe that toxic estrogens increased by environmental chemicals and pesticides are one major cause in the increase of certain cancers.

It would be wise to wear protection against pollution as well as a sunscreen. Some of us already wear patches to stop smoking or to absorb synthetic hormones or heart medications. Wouldn't it be great to wear a shield against pollution and allergies? Georgette Klinger's Prime Time Rebalancing Cream provides phytohormones from soy and yam, safe food sources of estrogen and progesterone. It's a light, moisturizing cream that softens the skin as it protects against irritation. It may not replace clean air, but it lets your skin feel fresh at any age.

Reduce Internal Inflammation

Skin sensitivity is far more complicated than exposure to pollution and ultraviolet rays. Corresponding to the current rise in skin cancer has been the increasing number of people who smoke, drink alcohol, and use birth control pills or irritating acne medicines. That and the sun makes an explosive combination of irritants!

Smoking irritates the lungs and concentrates toxins that harm the entire body. Chinese herbalists believe that smoking harms the skin. Medical and street drugs frequently constrict energy circulation or dehydrate. One of the best things we can do, aside from using a sunscreen and limiting sun exposure during peak midday hours, is to reduce impurities and inflammation so that the body can make new skin the way it is supposed to.

To help prevent conditions that could lead to cancers, add generous amounts of Asian medicinal mushrooms to your diet. Reishi+ liquid extract (ling zhi) made by Long Hay Flat and sold by www.eastearthtrade.com greatly increases energy and immunity to illness. Just 5–10 drops twice daily offer a faster, safer, and more effective stimulant than caffeine found in coffee or chocolate.

Treatment

Western Medical Approach

If you opt for Western medical treatment of spots, which in most cases means removal, you will need to make a distinction between plastic surgeons—skilled in surgery and sensitive to esthetics—and the regular medical generalist or dermatologist. When the reason you are consulting a skin specialist is beauty, consider your options carefully. Treatment generally costs more with a plastic surgeon, but it depends on where the spot is located.

Why spot removal and optional cosmetic surgery are not considered a health issue is beyond me; appearance greatly impacts on mood, energy, and general well-being. However, insurance coverage is limited. Costs and quality of service at clinics vary. Linking lifestyle habits to health and beauty concerns has led to lawsuits, notably against the cigarette industry. You may be paying the high price of your doctor's health insurance. At the same time, there exists a vast alternative medical establishment because medical treatments can be time-consuming, costly, and do not always yield aesthetically pleasing results. The beauty benefits of such an establishment have not been fully realized.

Chinese Medical Approach

Herbs that cleanse impurities, enhance blood, and promote circulation are recommended for improving skin quality. Often they can prevent further spots or eventually lighten freckles. Smokers and people who love spicy foods and alcoholic beverages, or who use medical and street drugs often report improvements in skin quality, luster, and texture after a few acupuncture treatments. The aim of acupuncture used to curb addictions is to help the body create new, healthy tissue inside and out. In the process, many underlying problems such as poor digestion and circulation can be improved.

Age Spots (Liver Spots)

While skin cancer can occur at any age, skin spots may be related to age. Harmless, rough, waxy brown or black spots, called seborrheic keratoses, may start appearing on skin just before midlife and become prevalent with age. Flat, brown spots that form after years of sun exposure—age spots, also called solar lentigines—are common in adults who have tanned or spent much time outdoors, and are said to be flat patches of increased pigmentation. The increased pigmentation may be brought on by aging, exposure to sun or other forms of ultraviolet light, or other unknown causes. Liver spots, which are extremely common after 55 years of age, occur most often on the backs of the hands and on the forearms, shoulder, face, and forehead. These are the areas of highest sun exposure.

Ask a dermatologist about liver spots and they will advise you to avoid the sun. Chinese herbalists say the spots are related to liver weakness and poor circulation. Perhaps the sun aggravates an underlying condition. In any case, it is wise to avoid foods and substances that might interfere with circulation and cause congestion or inflammation. They include cigarettes, alcohol, garlic, and spicy, hot, and fried foods.

Susan Lin's Beautiful Skin Tea

Susan Lin, owner of Lin Sisters Herb Shop in New York, recommends individualized teas for her customers. A daily tea for liver spots would contain blood-enhancing tonic herbs as well as herbs that increase circulation to heal the liver and skin—for example, equal parts of rehmannia, ligusticum, dong quai, red peony, lycium fruit, astragalus, cistanche, and peach seed (a moistening laxative). Simmer the ingredients for one hour and drink a cup between meals. Susan also sells the Yin/Yang Sisters instant beverages for a variety of conditions including problem skin. You can find her contact information in the Annotated Resource Guide at the end of this book.

Steamed tienchi is warming (for the spleen and pancreas in TCM) and stimulating for circulation and blood production. You might take ½ teaspoon of the powder in water daily or 3–9 tablets daily. If steamed tienchi makes you feel hot or dizzy, use raw tienchi ginseng, which is cooling. Both greatly stimulate circulation to help resolve bruises, swelling, pain, and internal bleeding. Men or women can use any of the above remedies for liver spots.

Freckles

The Miller-Keane Medical Dictionary defines freckles as benign, small, tan to brown macules occurring on sun-exposed skin, especially in children and tending to fade in adult life. Freckles resemble age spots, but they darken after exposure to sunlight, whereas lentigines do not.

One of my clients with pale skin, freckles, and cold hands said, "I get freckles that have nothing to do with the sun. When I am tired, my skin sometimes feels numb, cold, or as though something is crawling over it." Poor circulation can take many forms for men and women. Often it can be corrected with proper nutrition or a homeopathic mineral supplement. Homeopathic calc. phos. (calcium phosphate) 6x strength is recommended for poor nutrition because it is an important constituent of saliva and gastric juices. It promotes healthy organs, bones, and teeth. It improves blood production and makes blood coagulation possible. Lacking this form of calcium harms circulation.

As a beauty remedy, calc. phos. 6x strength is specifically recommended for freckles, a creepy-crawling sensation of the skin, or numbness that results from poor circulation. It is a fine restorative after illness and exhaustion. It is best to use it throughout the day at least five times under the tongue or in a little water. Avoid mixing it with food or drinks.

Daily Massage for Enhanced Circulation

The following massage promotes circulation and is useful for preventing nervous tension that may contribute to many chronic conditions, including age spots, anxiety, joint stiffness, insomnia, and depression. The massage, based on lymphatic drainage techniques and acupuncture theory, can be done anywhere. It works well in a soothing bath or as part of a facial.

Have on hand some fresh cold milk, ice cubes made from milk, fresh cucumber slices, or juiced cucumber. Coat your hands with a cooling oil such as sunflower, safflower, rapeseed, or olive oil. Massage your shoulders to release tightness. With your fingertips, stroke your neck upward from the base to the chin. Stroke upward on the cheeks to the temples. Tap lightly on the forehead to the temples, and the top of the cheekbones. Do not rub your eyes.

Press with your middle three fingertips at the outside of each nostril as you deeply inhale, then release as you exhale. Press the same way under the cheekbone towards your ears. Press your fingers all around your ears, in front and in back, as you inhale.

Massage your ears—front, sides, and back—using the cooling oil. This can release tension stored anywhere in the body. It may feel painful or odd because all acupuncture meridians pass through the ear to the brain. Your massage liberates circulation through the entire body. Acupuncture treatments used for addictions always treat the ear, because points used for internal organs are located on the ear's surface. Some areas may look red, irritated, crusty, or blemished or feel painful. Those represent areas of inflammation in the body.

You may want to gently bend your neck or make other subtle movements with your head and shoulders to adjust your circulation. It will feel good to move your shoulders in circles and then lift them to your ears and release. If you prefer, you can extend the massage to the hairline and head. After the massage, rinse face, neck, and ears with warm water. Soak a clean face cloth with cold milk or cucumber juice and apply it for five minutes to your face, neck, and chest. Rinse with cool water.

A Natural Spot Removal Solution

Commercial spot and wart removers are available in pharmacies. Most contain up to 17% salicylic acid, which is highly inflammatory and can temporarily increase skin redness or agitation.The results vary quite a bit depending on how well you heal. Brunettes and black-haired people with darker complexions have more myelin, a protein, in their bodies. The protein makes their scars look darker and thicker than for blondes. As a safe alternative, for everyday use, I combine pure essential lemon oil (an exfoliant) with a pleasant body oil or cream, for example Origins Gloom Away Grapefruit Body Gloss. The oils in the Gloom Away help the lemon oil penetrate to make a tingling exfoliant for face and body. Be careful when using exfoliants, natural or otherwise: avoid sensitive areas and broken capillaries.

The following information will be of interest whether or not you use a spot removal treatment. Medederma, a greaseless gel, lightens scars over time. Made in Germany for Merz Skin Care Products in Greensboro, North Carolina, it contains onion extract (*Alium cepa*). Onion is a blood cleanser and thinner when eaten. The gel is said to improve color and texture of scars resulting from surgery, injury, burns, acne, and stretch marks.

Sunscreens

Sunscreens of SPF 15 and higher are recommended for everyone. Being fair, I prefer one that is SPF 45 when exposed to midday or winter sun. High SPF sunscreens contain 5–10% or more titanium dioxide, a mineral used to create a physical barrier to block the sun's rays. When exposure is limited, I might use a moisturizer such as Weleda Diaper-Care, which contains zinc oxide 12%, almond oil, lanolin, hydrolyzed beeswax, and extracts of calendula and chamomile flowers, and has a natural, light fragrance. It is wasted on babies' bottoms! It smells nice and feels very soothing. Zinc oxide is the only truly natural (nonchemical) sunscreen.

A Sunshine Exfoliant Treatment

To turn your time in the sun into a beauty treatment, add a few drops of essential oil of lemon, a safe, natural exfoliant, to your sunscreen in order to refine your complexion. All exfoliants increase sun sensitivity, but oil of lemon is not as strong as other fruit acids. Natural oils in lemon protect the skin. Lemon contains vitamin C and is by nature cooling and healing.

Extra-Mild Products with Minimal Additives

Skin stress, such as breakouts, aging, and spots, is aggravated by the chemical additives, dyes, and alcohol-based perfumes added to beauty products.

The following brands omit animal ingredients and alcohol. They use pure, natural, organic plant extracts, oils, vitamins, enzymes, and the minimum amount of FDA-required preservatives. I am happy to highly recommend them.

Kiss My Face

As you will see in my Annotated Resource Guide beginning on page 238, I rave about the consistent high quality of Kiss My Face products. They make cleansers, moisturizers, shaving creams, toners, and most other beauty products for sensitive skin. I think their moisturizers and sunscreen products are particularly worth mentioning.

Protection with Added Color

Kiss My Face's tinted moisturizers are healthy makeup made with organic ingredients. The liquids cover blemishes with a base containing plant dyes, essential oils, and clay. Choose colors from a full spectrum of shades: Manilla, Beach, Sisal, Rattan, Clay, or Branch. You can apply them with or without moisturizers because the natural ingredients blend with your complexion type to form a shear mat finish used by men and women.

Kiss My Face makes an exciting line of sun-care products that include nonchemical sunblocks with oat protein complex for added moisture. Sun Swat is a sunblock with titanium dioxide (SPF 15) and a natural insect repellant made from citronella, pennyroyal, and other essential oils. They also make a nice After Sun Aloe Soother you apply after being in the sun too long. It contains soothing jewelweed and yucca as well as organic aloe. If you want to avoid the sun altogether, apply Kiss My Face Natural Instant Sunless Tanner with walnut extract and go nutty with a warm, glowing color.

Jason Natural Cosmetics

Most of us get our vitamin C from an orange or a pill. Jason's line of Ester C facial products include Super-C Cleanser, Toner, and Hyper-C Serum. All contain a nonirritating, antiinflammatory form of vitamin C known to reduce signs of aging and skin stress. Super-C Cleanser comes with a natural bristle brush for deeper cleansing. It is washed off with water and followed by Super-C Toner to refine large pores. Hyper-C Serum, applied twice daily, is heavier and oilier than a toner. Its rejuvenating ingredients include green tea, grapeseed extract, and antistress minerals.

If you prefer a light touch, Jason makes Aloe Vera Super Gel, a fresh, clean-smelling skin moisturizer with spirulina seaweed. It feels cool after a shave.

Burt's Bees

Burt's Bees Orange Essence Facial Cleanser removes "dirt, oil, makeup and pollutants while moistening the skin." The sweet orange, oil-rich ointment applied with the fingers and washed off with warm water contains vegetable glycerin, olive and orange oils, lanolin, beta-carotene and vitamin E, and rosemary extract.

Yummy smelling Carrot Nutritive Day Creme contains sunflower, wheat germ, avocado, grapeseed, carrot seed, and coconut oils, orange wax, vitamin E, rosemary extract, beta-carotene, and natural enzymes to repair and revive sun-damaged, aging skin. It penetrates, leaving a protective coating against wind and cold—and probably attracts rabbits.

Burt's Bees Garden Tomato Soap and Tomato Toner are lighter and less rich, for troubled complexions.

Herbal Bath Products

I like Kiss My Face bath and shower gels. Rough Thyme Shower Gel combines stimulating natural exfoliants bergamot, thyme, cinnamon, clove, and lemon to daily whisk off the layer of dead cells. You may prefer their Early to Bed Moisture Bath for relaxation. Clove and ylang ylang are quieting and warming, lavender soothes anxiety and restlessness, chamomile makes you feel closer to Mom, Neroli is aromatic and antiseptic, and jasmine is added just in case you wish you were soaking in a tropical jungle.

Kiss My Face Active Athletic Muscle Relaxant Bath contains eucalyptus, arnica, balm mint, chamomile, fennel, comfrey, ivy, juniper, and slippery elm in a base of witch hazel.

A Hypoallergic Deodorant with a Plus

Most natural brands make deodorants with safe natural ingredients such as baking soda, essential oils, or minerals found in nature. Jason's is the only company I have seen to include Chinese yam cream, recommended for menopausal complaints, in a daily roll-on deodorant. That is taking safety one giant step further.

Especially for Men

Jock itch is not limited to men, but the expression was born in their locker rooms. The red, itching rash in the body's creases is made worse from sweating. A fungus may require an antibiotic cream or tea tree oil in water, but for a simple heat rash, calamine lotion keeps skin dry and promotes healing. Homeopathic kali mur. 6x and silicea 6x taken orally several times daily between meals will slowly detoxify the body and help prevent or heal rashes. If the rash is red hot and burning, 5 pills of homeopathic belladonna 30C dissolved under the tongue several times daily between meals will help cool it.

Lola's Way

Skin brightness is closely related to circulation. You can start to improve ruddy or sallow skin today by adding ¼ teaspoon of tienchi ginseng powder to a cup of hot water or tea twice daily. For a ruddy complexion, hot flashes, or excess thirst, use Raw Tienchi Powder (cooling) to reduce inflammation and high cholesterol. For a sallow complexion, chills, and cold weather, use Steamed Tienchi Powder (warming) to enhance blood production. Both are beneficial for circulation to help prevent age spots.

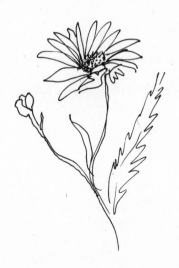

14

Your Best Face Forward

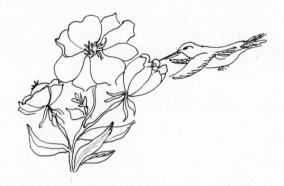

"To discern the beauty of a thing is the finest point
to which we can arrive. A colour-sense is more
important, in the development of the individual,
than a sense of right and wrong."
—OSCAR WILDE

What part of your beauty is art and what part nature? Makeup can enhance or hide the real you. Oscar Wilde, a classical scholar, poet, playwright, and dandy, insisted that art, not flesh, portrays reality. "Aesthetics make life lovely and wonderful, fill it with new forms, and give it progress, and variety and change," he writes in *Intentions,* a collection of his essays from 1891.

Chinese opera still uses thick makeup resembling a mask to identify characters. Since before the Song dynasty (960–1279), the traditional makeup immediately informed the audience about a character's importance and intentions. Wicked characters wear white face: Cao Cao has a dagger painted on his white forehead to signify evil intentions behind an insidious smile. Yellow expresses cruelty: Wang Liao is witty and ruthless. Green indicates loyalty; blue mightiness; and purple honesty. Gold and silver makeup designate gods and demons. In Chinese opera, every rung of society is expressed with makeup.

In the West, mega-stars like James Dean and Marilyn Monroe became icons. We copy their haircuts, makeup, and style whether it suits us or not. In this book, I stress the importance of creating a *personal* aesthetic. Your face can express any aspect of your personality. Does your face reflect your current needs?

A Style Mask

Have you used the same facial products and makeup for the past 10 or more years? That turns your beauty into a mask. Art may be eternal, but beauty products should not be. Ignoring complexion changes is hazardous to your looks. As we age, skin texture and coloring change. We need to be sensitive to our skin, the largest organ of respiration and detoxification. This chapter covers healthy facial treatments to protect beauty and makeup application that work wonders. In treating the two topics simultaneously, we take inspiration from the work of Georgette Klinger, known as "the Dean of Skin Care." She believes the basis of facial beauty to be healthy, clean skin.

Applying safe, effective beauty products especially chosen to enhance your particular skin type and treat your current skin condition is one important way to ensure healthy beauty. The right products allow your skin to breathe, relax, and rejuvenate. That concept seems obvious to us now. However, it was an innovation at the beginning of this century, when women painted their faces with lead-based paint and ate chalk for a bright complexion. Our current ideas on clean and healthy skin had their birth in Eastern Europe.

Georgette Klinger, now in her 90s, was in her teens when she won a beauty contest in her native Czechoslovakia. The prize, an elaborate set of makeup and skin-care products, made her skin break out. Because of that, she studied with leading dermatologists in Europe and devoted the rest of her life to skin care.

After fleeing Nazi occupation in Czechoslovakia, she opened the first American skin-care salon in New York in 1941. Ms. Klinger is exemplary among that generation of women, including Helena Rubinstein, Elizabeth Arden, Estee Lauder, and Mary Kay, who became titans of the beauty industry. Often they came from poor backgrounds and built their companies by paying personal attention to every detail. Mary Kay and Avon gave women direct experience in sharing in enormous profits. Beauty, more than a means to personal satisfaction, made that generation of independent businesswomen rich and famous. Mary Kay never forgot her secret of success—the importance of being feminine. The caring attitude expressed by their organizations remains a vital part of the beauty business. At Georgette Klinger, Inc., beauty experts educate their clients about how to care for their skin. Ms. Klinger, who has a lovely complexion with invisible pores, is fond of saying, "If you are blessed with beautiful skin you have to keep it up. For problematic skin, you have to work harder."

The Salon Experience

If you would rather buy a toy for your house, car, or kids than pamper yourself with a monthly salon facial, you are missing a golden opportunity for rejuvenation and quiet reflection. I offer the following vicarious treat to tired, overworked men and women of all ages. I might have chosen Avon's luxurious Fifth Avenue Spa or a European equivalent, but for sentimental reasons, I chose Georgette Klinger on Madison Avenue because it is like a trip home. The aestheticians from Russia, Ukraine, Poland, Hungary, and Czechoslovakia incorporate the most advanced skin-care methods in a serene and nurturing environment. Their treatments are personalized, highly professional, and motherly.

Any serious attempt to enhance face, neck, and decolletage beauty includes cleansing, toning, and rejuvenating facial treatments as well as makeup. Just as in fashion modeling, where the right undergarments bring out clothes' design, a facial is the first step to externally protect, beautify, and prepare the skin for makeup. If you are going to take a jet somewhere, appear on television, conduct a business meeting; if you are sick or need to have an operation; if a friend has arranged a date for you to meet someone new—have a professional facial. It will calm your nerves and rejuvenate your skin. Stress is dehydrating for the body and especially for the skin. A salon facial once a month can help prevent signs of aging.

Georgette Klinger's Nine-Step Facial

Most beauty salons offer facials. Georgette Klinger salons offer highly individualized treatments and products according to your skin type. In New York or one of their eight locations across the United States, Georgette Klinger's is a great place to get a revitalizing beauty and energy lift! My facialist, Sara, who is from Moscow, applied Georgette Klinger products for my skin type. The facial included:

- Makeup removal with a light, nonscented makeup remover chosen for my skin type
- Close-up facial examination to see individual problems
- A facial massage with a lightweight, nonscented cream
- Facial steam with a delicious, freshly made chamomile tea
- Deep pore cleansing to remove impurities
- A facial mask made of almond, oatmeal, and honey, which smells good enough to eat

- A mask containing vitamin C and green tea to help tone the skin
- A cool, revitalizing facial mask
- A moisturizing hand treatment

As I drifted into nirvana, Sara applied a moisture cream to my hands and arms to the elbow. She slipped my hands into electrically warmed gloves for extra moisture penetration. I mentally made a list of people to whom I would to give this Nine Step Facial treatment as a gift.

My new at-home beauty routine especially designed for me by the staff at Georgette Klinger uses products that contain no drying alcohol or chemical fragrance. After cleansing and toning my skin, I especially enjoy applying Georgette Klinger's Skin Booster with Vitamin C. It glides on silky smooth. I use it to lightly massage my neck and face with upward strokes— a skin treat.

An Individualized Facial for the Change of Seasons

In Chapter 4, I recommended seasonal foods for lasting skin beauty. When my tan begins to fade; when the city's bustling drains me; when rich diet, pollution, or weather changes bring on skin stress and blemishes, I have a deep-cleansing and balancing treatment. One good example is Georgette Klinger's 12-phase Virtual Perfection facial. This one-hour treatment is customized for each person's individual needs, but always includes a thorough cleansing step and creams and lotions to nourish and protect the skin and leave it glowing and vibrant. In addition to the antiaging, antioxidant benefits of green tea and the skin restructuring power of alpha and beta hydroxy fruit acids, all Virtual Perfection formulas include ginkgo biloba extract, mineral-rich sea algae, nourishing, moistening oat extract, and vitamins A, C, and E.

After cleansing, followed by an in-depth skin analysis to determine the skin's condition, an alpha-beta hydroxy skin lotion is used to exfoliate the skin, gently remove damaged surface cells, and prepare the skin for the benefits of the Virtual Perfection ingredient complex. A 15-minute massage with green tea cream is used to relax and tone the face, throat, and decolletage. That releases pressure and stress from facial muscles. Then an aromatic steam treatment with green teas envelop the skin and prepare it for more deep pore cleansing.

Two Virtual Perfection masks follow. In the first, the skin basks in a freshly prepared herbal pack combined with blended green teas that hydrate and leave the skin feeling smooth, supple, and totally comfortable. During this mask, Virtual Perfection Body Moisturizer is massaged from fingertips to elbows. Green tea is also an important ingredient in the second Virtual Perfection Mask B, a cool gel formula that is used over the face, eye area, throat, and decolletage. This soothing mask minimizes fine lines, redness, and puffiness and leaves the skin smooth, nourished, and refreshed.

A revitalizing mist of Virtual Perfection Toning Lotion combines, among others, lavender extract, algae, watercress, St. John's wort, and green tea to stimulate complexion renewal with soothing orchid, calendula, camomile, and elderflower extracts in cooling witch hazel extract. A nourishing application of Virtual Perfection Face Cream completes the session.

Georgette Klinger's facials and makeup consultations involve a detailed analysis of individual skin type. From the point of view of alternative health and beauty care, I appreciate their personalized care. Appropriate products are chosen from among hundreds of Georgette Klinger products in order to match your needs. Their Bulgarian-born director of skin-care training, Astrid Bedrossian, once told me, "Our products are so natural that one mask comes from a lake in Europe."

Skin Stress from Pollution and Smoking

If you live in a city or smoke, you have *aging* skin no matter what your age. For delicate, mature skin; for skin that is withered from sun damage, hormone imbalances, or TV studio lights; and for anyone who smokes, extra lubrication and protection is needed from rich nourishing creams. Georgette Klinger's Prime Time or Chamomile Cream reduce skin stress. Klinger's Advanced Oxygen Moisture Cream adds protection from oxygen in peroxide. Skin Booster with Vitamin C, a silky moisturizer in a pump bottle, goes on smooth as it nourishes with vitamins, antioxidants, and ceramides to brighten, nourish and firm skin. Georgette Klinger's Eye Cream 2 combines lanolin, castor oil, wheat germ oil, rose hip seed oil, avocado and sesame oil to minimize fine lines and wrinkles.

Home Facials Then and Now

Nineteenth-century stage actress Adah Isaacs Menken's death-defying role as Mazeppa gave her international stardom. Playwright and journalist Charles Reade described her complexion as whitened with lead paint. Menken's makeup was vital. The darling of Civil War America was secretly a woman of color from New Orleans. Menken died at the top of her fame in her thirties, probably from tuberculosis and lead makeup poisoning. Her idol, Lola Montez, recommended natural beauty treatments, not cover makeup.

Lola's most amusing facial treatment is high protein: "I knew many fashionable ladies in Paris who used to bind their faces, every night on going to bed, with thin slices of raw beef, which is said to keep the skin from wrinkles, while it gave a youthful freshness and brilliancy to the complexion." I imagine it also attracted flies. For a dose of facial protein, I would rather mix pineapple juice with pure egg protein powder to make a thick paste and apply it for no longer than 20 minutes as a complexion-refining mask.

A mask Lola recommended "when dimness and wrinkles of age are extinguishing the roses of youth" is credited to Madam Vestris. It contained "the whites of four eggs boiled in rose-water, an ounce of alum, half an ounce of oil of sweet almonds." First, beat the ingredients together until it assumes the consistency of a paste, then spread the paste on to a silk or muslin mask to be worn all night. I guess you have to sleep alone when using this contraption.

Origins Charcoal Mask or Georgette Klinger's Deep Pore Cleansing Mask are easier and nicer to use. The latter's ingredients include almond meal, kaolin clay, honey, bitter almond oil, iron oxides, and talc.

Facial Washes and Toners

Lola's favorite simple recipes for facial washes include brandy and rose water. Another one, from France, used pumpkin, a natural exfoliant. The ingredients were: "equal parts of pumpkin seeds, pumpkin (a natural exfoliant), and cucumber, pounded til reduced to powder. Then add sufficient fresh cream to dilute the flour and to make paste. Add a grain of musk and a few drops of oil of lemon. Leave on for 20–30 minutes or overnight. Wash off with warm water. It gives a remarkable purity and brightness to the complexion."

A pumpkin pie in the face is messy. A better option is Pumpkin Exfoliating Mask made by Zia Natural Skincare. Zia's Pumpkin Exfoliating Mask delivers 100 nutrients to the skin. Fran Strachan, founder and president of Zia Natural Skincare, believes that for skin to look good the ingredients have to be healthy.

A Kiss for Everyone

If you insist on beauty products that are natural, organic, and cruelty-free without animal ingredients, artificial colors, and unnecessary chemicals, Kiss My Face is your best choice on the health-food store level. For morning-fresh cleansing, Kiss My Face Citrus Cleanser with lemon, lime, and olive oils, aloe vera, and other herbs, flowers, and vitamins is a light cream for all skin types (and can be washed off with water). Citrus Essence Astringent, a spray for oily and combination skin types, blots excess oil and unclogs pores. It tones and purifies without drying alcohol. The natural citrus fragrance lets you start the day with a smile.

Are you wondering what to give the one you love, the person who has everything, including you? Give a Kiss home facial. See www.kissmyface.com for details.

- Remove makeup with Kiss Organics Shea Butter Eye Make Up Remover.

- Cleanse with Kiss Organics Gentle Face Cleanser for dry skin or Kiss Organics Foaming Facial Cleanser for oily skin.
- Massage Kiss Organics Organic & Jojoba Mint Scrub over face and neck. Rinse with warm water.
- Spray Kiss Organics Aloe & Chamomile Toner for dry skin or Kiss Organics Aloe & Tea tree Astringent for oily or combination skin.
- Dab Kiss Organics A, C, & E Eye Opener on sensitive skin below eyes.
- Apply Kiss Organic Botanical Acne Gel to troubled areas.
- Apply over entire face and neck Kiss Organics Lemongrass Souffle Masque for dry skin or Kiss Organics Deep Pore Masque for oily skin.
- Saturate two cotton balls with Aloe & Chamomile Toner and place over eyes. Lie flat with your feet up for 20 minutes.
- Massage onto shoulders, hands, and feet Kiss Organics Ester C Body Lotion. Rinse with warm water, splash with cold water, and spray with toner.

Follow with serums and moisturizers for your skin type:

- Dry skin: first apply Kiss Organics Anti Ox or Ester C Serum, then Kiss Organics C & A Ultra Rich Moisturizer.
- Oily skin: Kiss Organics Anti Ox Serum, then Kiss Organics Ultra Light Facial Creme.
- Blemished skin: First Kiss Organics Anti-Ox Serum and Botanical Acne Gel, then Kiss Organics Ultra Light Moisturizer.
- Reapply A, C & E Eye Opener to under-eye area.

Facial Aromatherapy

Ancient Egyptians used resins such as pine, myrrh, and frankincense for the care of skin and scalp. For our use, they are disinfectant, drying, and healing to wounds. Myrrh reverses spoilage. Frankincense (boswellia) from Somalia and India has become recognized as a pain treatment for tired muscles and arthritis. Frankincense stirs circulation and helps to dissolve impurities.

When using pure essential oil of myrrh and frankincense as part of a facial treatment, add a few drops to water for a facial steam. You can add them to your favorite moisture cream or lotion. To increase local blood circulation and enliven a sallow complexion, apply a few drops of the essential oils to a moisture lotion as a stimulating skin treatment. Avoid sensitive areas and rinse off myrrh and frankincense with warm water after waiting up to one hour. It feels like a calm walk on a clear day. If you have a dull complexion, shortness of breath, pallor, fatigue, or you smoke, your skin and—for lack of better words—*aura* need this.

Natural Exfoliation

Exfoliation or mild peeling is strongly recommended by beauty and health experts to prevent dry, crusty, or aging skin. Instead of using harsh chemicals on elbows, knees, and feet, try a natural scrub made of oil and salt such as Origins Soft Rub or one that you make at home using Epsom salts, sunflower oil, and your favorite essential oils. For a moisturizing scrub, you will need to use richer ingredients. For example, Zia makes a Brown Sugar Body Polish for a sweet alternative to salt scrubs.

Unless you have an ultrasensitive complexion, facial cleansing grains are recommended daily or three times weekly to remove flaky, dead skin. Cornmeal made into a watery paste has been used by herbalists. Zia's Citrus Night Time Reversal cream is nice because it refines your skin while you sleep. Citrus is digestive for dead skin, stimulating for new skin growth, and a source of useful oils and nutrients.

Bathtub Facial Exercises

These movements energize the muscles that shape your face. Avoid doing them in public or you will be taken for a nut! Squeeze all your features together at the tip of your nose as though your entire face comes to a point. Hold for the count of 10 as you breath normally. Release and relax your face and repeat it several times. Now, do the opposite: open your eye, nose and mouth wide and stick our your tongue like a roaring lion.

To firm your forehead, place your fingertips on your eyebrows as though to keep them from moving. Lift up your brow against the resistance. Tap very lightly on the sides and top of your head with your fingertips to bring more circulation to the areas that lift your face. ·

Makeup Art

Makeup holds a magic fascination recognized since the ancient Egyptians. Paintings and sculptures of famously beautiful Queen Nefertiti dating from the Amarna period (c. 1352–1336 B.C.) clearly show her eye makeup, cheek rouge, and lip paint colors. The queen's black eyeliner, made from galena, a gray lead ore from Upper Egypt, extends the length of her large eyes. Green eye paint made from malachine, a carbonate of copper, was also popular. Visit the great Egyptian collections at New York's Metropolitan Museum of Art, Cairo's Egyptian Museum, or Oxford's Ashmolean Museum, and you will find cosmetic palettes and paraphernalia used to grind eye and face powders as well as mirrors with which to view the results. Makeup was—and remains—one of the essential ways that humans communicate sexuality.

Egyptian men and women wore eye makeup to indicate their social status and sexual appeal. Applying it daily was considered a ritual offering to the gods. A mummy mask from the 18th Dynasty (c. 1550–1295 B.C.) found in Musees Royaux d'Art et d'Histoire in Brussels shows a prosperous young man whose elaborate eye and eyebrow paint give him attractive androgynous features. Makeup, part of an elaborate offering of wealth and beauty, allowed the gods to judge the dead person's importance and soul.

What Makeup Says About You

Gad Cohen, a style genius whose work we will study in the following chapter, believes that the most beautiful faces look natural and relaxed. The purpose of makeup is to create harmony." Does your makeup enhance or hide you? Does your face show others who you are, who you could be, or who you wish you were? Applied in ignorance, makeup easily becomes an object of ridicule. Used with skill, makeup brings out the depths, value, and art in you.

Simone de Beauvoir was critical of fashion and cosmetics throughout most of the second chapter of *The Second Sex,* volume two. Her so-called bible of postwar feminism was conceived in humble circumstances—a modest hotel room overlooking a neighborhood bistro where she and Sartre discussed philosophy and verbally dissected a selection of shared female lovers. The two seduced and subsequently abandoned several such "objects." Momentarily setting cunning aside, de Beauvoir suggests a deeper significance of making up when she writes, "To care for her beauty, to dress up, is a kind of work that enables (a woman) to take possession of her person, as she takes possession of her home through housework, her persona then seems chosen and created by herself."

Most of the time, we don't consider applying makeup to be an existential act of self-creation. We wear it because it is an enjoyable part of dressing. Makeup makes us look and feel better. Dr. Vernon Coleman, in *Face Values: How the Beauty Industry Affects You,* suggests that women apply makeup daily as a mood changer.

Your Face as Art

One of the best ways to get a correct, objective view of how you really look is by having a consultation with a top-drawer makeup artist. A beauty expert, experienced with models, executives, politicians, and celebrities, can appraise your style and beauty products as well as offer suggestions on how to bring your look up to date. The best makeup artists are sensitive communicators, who take the time and care needed to make you look and feel fabulous. Based on their experience with many clients, they can advise you on how to bring out your best gifts in order to accomplish what you want.

Your Natural Healthy Coloring

Before you decide the colors for your makeup palette, you need to establish your natural healthy coloring. Age, chemical pollution, smoking, bad diet, and stress can leave you looking ashen, jaundiced, pale, ruddy, or some other unhealthy hue. Your natural skin and hair colors are what you were born with and how you would look in perfect health. Some stylists examine your hand color in order to choose the best shade for makeup foundation. They look at your eyes for eye-shadow color. They might ask about your childhood hair color. Healthy skin is moist and has a fine texture, good tone, and healthy natural color. You fix up best if you look healthy under makeup. Thick makeup, like a Chinese opera mask, looks fake and increases a wrinkled appearance.

A Chinese doctor notices facial hue to ascertain energy level, circulation, and general health. The following chart summarizes their energetic approach:

Natural Skin Color or Hue	Problem	Requires
Pale or ashen skin	Weak adrenal energy	Use tonic herbs (see Chapter 3) Skin products that contain Vitamin C and antioxidants
Jaundice (yellow or bronze hue)	Liver health	Eat low-fat, cleansing diet Use skin products that are moderately rich, not oily
Ruddy complexion, facial broken capillaries	Sensitive skin Exposure to harsh weather Hormone imbalance	Avoid stimulants (caffeine), harsh climate, and spices; Use alcohol-free, nourishing products for fragile skin

Choosing a Makeup Artist

It is important to choose a sensitive stylist to advise you about color and design. You don't want to look like this month's fashion statement, whether you like it or not. Besides, so much of makeup is subjective. A stylist can create a grand illusion or a big mistake with a slight of hand.

Clif deRaita, Georgette Klinger's National Director of Makeup, aims to bring out the best natural features, coloring, and style integrity you have to offer. He analyzes your natural coloring by looking at your eyes or by asking about your childhood hair color. Then he chooses colors, as a painter would, to enhance your natural gifts. Clif told me, "I come from an artistic family that stressed painting. As a child, I did watercolors of women's eyes and swans. Now," he smiles, "I paint women's eyes, making them into swans." Clif danced for years on Broadway with Bob Fosse. He is slim, animated, and light on his feet as does your makeup. He stands close, while you sit on a stool, and carefully demonstrates how to apply eye creams, liners, mascara, and the works. His celebrity clients need to look their best at all times.

How to Hide Fatigue

"It is difficult to completely hide fatigue," says Clif. "But there are some tricks you can do. When you are tired, that is not the time to apply more makeup. You have to deemphasize problem areas." Clif works with television anchor people or media personalities who may need to cover signs of stress. He suggests, "First thing in the morning, don't emphasize the lower eyelid. To draw the viewers' eye away from dark circles, curl the eyelashes to give the eye a lift."

Clif has deep-set, attractive, Mediterranean eyes to match his Italian olive complexion. He uses the size, shape, and color of glasses to deemphasize the lower lid. His small glasses fit right over his eyelids and do not extend over the eye area. The tops of the frames have a fine line of color but the lower part near the lower lid is clear with no frame. That deaccentuates the under-eye area.

Have Beauty, Will Travel

Jet travel presents extraordinary challenges. With Clif deRaita's help, you can design your personalized travel beauty kit. At Georgette Klinger, Inc., you cannot get product recommendations over the phone. You need to have a personalized facial consultation and treatment. However, I asked Clif about special problems faced by people during travel. He suggested creams you might use to turn an otherwise white-knuckle flight into a beauty retreat.

The following outline is organized according to weather conditions and skin type. For example, if you live or plan to fly to cold weather or if your skin is dry or mature, your beauty and makeup regime will differ from one required for hot weather, oily skin, or acne.

When I asked which products are most important to pack for traveling, Clif didn't hesitate: "Cleansing is the most important thing you can do for your skin. You need to use the right cleansing product suited to your skin type. It especially has to contain the right strength of cleansing ingredients. That's the most important. Many over-the-counter products are so harsh and drying that they require additional moisturizing. Many people have combination skin and need to moisturize only the neck, sides of the face, and above the mouth, not the chin and nose."

Cold Weather or Fragile, Dry, or Mature Skin

Use a mild cleansing lotion and wear a heavy, lubricating moisturizer during cold weather to reduce dryness, skin stress, and nerve sensitivity. A ruddy complexion, rosacea, parched skin, and neuralgia are aggravated because cold weather reduces circulation and energy. Typically, a person with hypothermia, a dangerously low body temperature, feels weak. Avoid this by drinking cinnamon tea to increase sweating and circulation. To prevent moisture and body heat from escaping, wear a protective coating of a heavy moisture cream to counter the weakening effects of cold.

Jet travel presents a perfect opportunity for a deep-nourishing facial treatment. Unless you expect a photo-op upon arrival, why wear makeup? It is better to coat yourself with a moisture barrier to prevent in-flight skin stress. For irritated or delicate skin, Georgette Klinger's Chamomile Cream is soothing. The natural flower fragrance is relaxing. For a dull or sallow complexion, Klinger's Advanced Oxygen Moisturizer contains antioxidant vitamins, soy protein, and various oils, including orange, corn, and jojoba, to protect and nourish the skin. The added oxygen from hydrogen peroxide, a main ingredient in this lotion, will be devoured by undernourished skin.

A rich skin cream massaged into hands and feet is more than a beauty treatment in cold weather. It will protect you from aches, aging, and energy loss. A rich oil-based cream outside can keep you warm inside. For downhill skiing or any exposure to drying, cold air, Clif advises wearing a facial cream such as Georgette Klinger's Sea Extracts Moisturizer. It combines sea vitamins, minerals, phytohormones, amino acids, and trace minerals. A rich treatment that protects sensitive eye tissue is Eye Cream #2, which combines lanolin, wheat germ oil, sesame oil, and avocado oil. Clif says, "Downhill skiing weakens the skin." He explained that skiing involves cold wind brushing against the face and extreme temperatures, which can encourage rosacea.

For rosacea, Clif recommends Georgette Klinger's Rosewater Spray, made from real petals imported from Bulgaria, which corrects skin pH balance after using water. It rehydrates the skin. Green tea and chamomile tea steams or splashed on will also calm the skin.

Before your trip or regularly during cold weather, Georgette Klinger recommends a protective facial treatment to prepare the skin for the change in climate. After the treatment, they recommend the right mask to take along with you. It may be their Moisture Recovery Dry Skin Mask or Polyplant Mask—both great ways to nourish your skin. If you normally exfoliate the skin, do it very gently in cold weather. Avoid alpha hydroxy acid treatments if your skin is irritated.

Winter Makeup

For cold, dry weather, use a makeup foundation that contains oil for extra richness. The color will be lighter than one you use in summer. For example, use colors ranging from Sunny Beige to Warm Ivory. If your skin is naturally sallow or pale, avoid yellow hair colors. When your hair and skin are the same tone, you fade into the wallpaper. A cool hair color will bring out the natural pink tones of your skin. Use lipstick and eye colors that are soft and rosy.

Hot Weather, Oily Skin, or Acne

Use a stronger cleansing lotion and exfoliant products in hot weather to help the skin breathe. Darker, thicker, or oily skin requires lighter moisturization and stronger cleansing products. If your skin is dry and sensitive, avoid products that contain alcohol, but steam your face with chamomile or green tea. Splash your face often with strained, cool green tea to protect complexion from sun damage. Its antioxidants prevent skin aging and dryness. Tea that has been steeped for more than 20 minutes has increased tannic acids that help to prevent skin burns.

Use cleansing grains or a cleanser that is removed with water such as Georgette Klinger's One Step Cleanser or Wash Off Cream. Pat the skin dry with a clean towel and apply a light moisturizer that contains green tea and aloe vera. Green tea protects your skin from pollution and sun damage, and aloe is soothing. Georgette Klinger's line of Virtual Perfection products, which contain fruit-based exfoliants and ginkgo extract are well suited to problem skin and exposure to pollution and stress. You can use exfoliant products daily and still keep your suntan. In fact, alpha and beta hydroxy acids in Virtual Perfection cleansers and creams can even out your color as they nourish your skin. For mature skin, Klinger's Prime Time Rebalancing Cream brings moisture and oxygen to the skin and Anti-Aging Lip Treatment prevents lipstick smears.

Suntan and Makeup

Clif advised me, "For a summer tan, use a creamy under-eye concealer that is dark enough to match your tan." Georgette Klinger's new Take Cover Eyelid Foundation works wonders. Blend the concealer with foundation to match your tan or natural dark color. Clif prefers a synthetic brush because it gives better control of the concealer.

For blendability and coverage, apply your foundation with a damp sponge using downward stokes. Light complexions can use warm, honey-beige tones—not pink—for summer or hot weather. Pinks and reds make blemishes more outstanding. Use an oil-free foundation in summer to avoid clogging pores. Clif advised me, "Keep your eye colors soft with a blonde powder for eyebrows, and enhance your lips with summer colors such as vibrant 'tangelo' and 'bitter/sweet' to match summer clothing colors."

Humidity and Pollution

Humid weather and pollution clog the skin pores and slow the body's natural cleansing process. A rainy day or a long plane ride can lead to unwanted water retention in your body, and bags of water under your eyes. It presents a good time to step up your internal cleansing routine. To protect your skin from environmental pollution, step up your internal consumption and external application of antioxidants such as green tea, amla, and vitamin C.

Makeup Style and The Inner You

Narcissus is not the only one who dreams of perfection. What if you have a secret or ideal self you want to indulge? When I shut my eyes and think about my beauty persona, I don't see a doctor at all. I see Greta Garbo, Ginger Rogers, Lana Turner, Carole Lombard, or other slinky movie actresses from the 1930s and 1940s. The appearance of the nonpublic you is as vital as your work persona, because it is the self reflected in Narcissus' pool. It is the person (or energy) you long to become. Tell your stylist about that image. Collect pictures of it to work from.

If you are not in touch with your style, ask some experts for their opinions. It takes courage and an open mind. For example, I once asked an Equity executive, who deals with actors daily, which actress *type* I am. You might ask a director what character you could play in a theater piece or what product you might sell in a commercial. I once asked a television producer what age she thought I could pass for. She replied, "In Hollywood, no one is over 35!" Ask your stylist, acting teachers, or vocal coach—not close friends or family—about your style or the impression you give. Their response may surprise you: they may not see your cherished self at all. It may be trapped under a layer of self doubt and neglect. A change in makeup and hairstyle can inspire you. Why not experiment? Try on wigs and clothes in colors you normally avoid. Compare your findings with style advice in the following chapter.

A Quick Fix

Need a two-minute makeover after a sleepless night? Wash with Georgette Klinger's cool blue One Step Cleanser. Splash on Kewra Water from India or Florida Water, which is used in Latin America and Asia. Spicy fragrance awakens your senses. Keep them in the refrigerator.

Blast away sinus congestion or sinus headache, clear your eyes, and bring a natural glow to your face with one drop of Australian Tea Tree Oil on a Q-tip gently swabbed in your nose. Dynamite!

Makeup to Minimize Wrinkles and Blemishes

- Apply a moisturizer appropriate for your skin type.
- Cover blemishes with a "neutralizer" (under-foundation color). Green

masks redness and capillaries. A white, pearled base covers scars and wrinkles. Orange covers blue or black.

- Apply a moderate coverage foundation with a semi-matte finish.
- Powder Blushers conceal dilated capillaries on the nose and cheeks.
- For ruddy or sallow skin, a water-based, high-oil color wash can be worn under foundation.
- Facial powder reflects light and minimizes wrinkles except for dry skin.
- Cream eye shadows minimize lines. Shiny powders are best suited for night.
- Apply Anti-Aging Lip Treatment by Georgette Klinger.
- An emollient-based lipstick is moistening. Matte lipsticks work for young skin.

Especially for Men

Makeup and body wraps, like plastic surgery, are becoming commonplace for men. Kiss My Face has a line of attractive tinted moisturizers that are appropriate for either sex. Clif deRaita told me, "We are all working longer hours. Some of us have shorter work weeks but still work longer hours. Men are using concealers to cover up dark circles under the eyes. They need to look healthier, especially in New York, because the job market is so competitive."

As the possibility of toxic pollution continues to threaten more than complexion, some informed people are seeking intense skin protection. A good area for a little well-placed New Narcissism is your skin. It absorbs everything, including pollution and toxic chemicals. Natural beauty products manufacturers would do well to create protective makeup. Here is my example:

Our first introduction to James Bond in the 1957 novel *From Russia With Love* is a photograph in which he is described as "handsome and ruthless." Secret agents have beauty secrets too. In Chapter 11, he awakens bored. After doing 20 slow press-ups followed by straight leg-lifts until his stomach muscles scream, and then touching his toes 20 times, he does arm and chest exercises combined with deep breathing until he is dizzy. He takes a very hot then cold shower and shaves. He is about to pull on a sleeveless, dark blue Sea Island cotton shirt and navy-blue tropical worsted trousers, and slip his bare feet into black leather sandals when—Whammy! That is the moment to apply a super-protective aftershave with sunscreen and suntan tint—makeup for machos.

Lola's Way

Lola was vehemently opposed to makeup, which she called "paints and powders." She found facial expression and a display of emotions to be more appealing. Her diatribe from *The Art of Beauty* includes, "A violently rouged woman is a disgusting sight . . . a distortion of nature's harmony!" She advised women to avoid foundation and apply a light vegetable rouge, which left most of the face as well as the neck and arms their natural color.

My vegetable suggestion is a dab of beet juice thinned with water on each cheek Cherry or berry juice feel and smell nice, but the color fades. For a subtle, transparent makeup look, blend several shades of powder blush. Smile broadly with your mouth closed, and then dab a circle of light-colored blush on either side of your nose. Blend it upward along the top of the cheek bone and use a darker tint in the cheek hollow. Cover both with a pale or shimmering loose powder.

If makeup, clothing color, and design choices for a personalized fashion statement remain a mystery, three style experts will guide you in the following chapter.

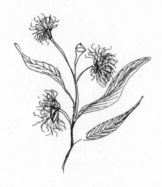

15

Style Genius

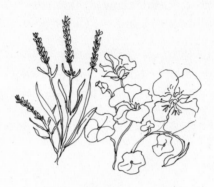

"Style is self-expression."
—MICHAEL FOSTER

Once, as a student in Paris, I snuck into the *pret-a-porter* fall fashion collections show. It was the year Yves St. Laurent had designed vivid red, green, and white gypsy-inspired puffy sleeves and wide, cheerful skirts. They were ravishing and joyous. The mood of world events and of fashion have never been the same. The collection heralded an exuberance that led to the fat 1980s. But by 1990, St. Laurent's lines were spare gray and navy-blue stovepipes inspired by the buildings and thoroughfares of New York, which he called the capital of the world. Fashion transcends design to mark the temperament of the times.

In this chapter, several top stylists, two men from New York and one woman from Los Angeles, will help you choose the colors and lines that work best for you no matter what the fashion trend.

Gad Cohen: "Style Is Not About Fashion."

Gad Cohen, who you met earlier, reminds me of the French screen idol Belmondo. His chiseled features and dark, tight-fitting, custom-made suit show off a slender, lithe frame. He is elegant and slightly *mechant* when he says, "I thinks it's interesting to be good but to always keep a little mischief in your style. Too good or too serene is flat; too crazy is also boring. You want to create excitement with your look."

With ultraprofessional cool, he glances at you, a lightbulb goes off in his head, and suddenly he dives in to create your look. You hold your breath and trust. His style sense and hair and makeup color genius have worked for models and actors known worldwide for their beauty. Fashion editors from *Vogue, Harpers Bazaar, Mademoiselle, Glamour, Elle,* and *Cosmopolitan* trust Gad. Glenn Close, Cindy Crawford, Barbra Streisand, Christy Turlington, and the like call on him to prepare for photo-ops. His style-savvy goes back lifetimes. Once in his apartment I admired a bust of Queen Nefertiti that Gad had sculpted as a child.

Gad agrees with Lola Montez and the natural school of beauty: "Bring out the best of what you have, but don't let it compete with your persona," says Gad. "Beauty is not necessarily style. Style can be impeccable taste. But you should always see the person, not the clothes." He believes that people can develop their unique style using a mirror. "If you have a large waist," he says, "play up your neck, shoulders, and legs. You have to deemphasize problems to make your body look the best you can."

Draw a Cross

As an exercise, take a recent photo of yourself looking forward with your head straight. Draw one line starting from the hairline down to the chin and another across the center of the eyes. How symmetrical are your features? Irregularity can be beautiful! What are your best features?

As an experiment, draw different shapes, colors, and sizes for your eyes, nose, mouth, chin, and hair. Gad believes, "Everybody has something about their looks that they like. They have to bring that out. There is no right or wrong about size, shape, and color. But you may want to deemphasize some things and emphasize others. If your lips are thin, play up your eyes. Make them more beautiful. Bangs can work like eyebrows to emphasize the eyes and reshape the face."

Everyone is asymmetrical. One side of our body does not match the other. Gad says, "The incredibly beautiful people are more symmetrical. Makeup is used to create symmetry." His clients Ashley Judd and Isabella Rossellini have elegant, balanced features. Using the cross method above, compare your features to beautiful people that you admire. When using makeup, emphasize the beauty that is naturally yours.

Hair Genius

Born in Montreal to a dynasty of haircutters that reaches back to Morocco, Gad loves to color and cut hair. In Chapter 10, we learned how to renew and protect hair from stress naturally. Hair is also a key element of style because it surrounds the face, shapes the head, and influences your height. The right hair color and style can be the first step in coordinating your makeup and clothing choices. Gad says, "You know that you have a flattering hair color if you look good without a tan. If you need to apply makeup to look better, your hair color is wrong. The right hair color works like makeup for your skin." For example, a yellow or sallow complexion often looks best with cool hair tones. Touch up a few strands in your hairline to let the flattering color reflect on your face.

A pleasing contrast is always a good idea. If complexion and hair color are exactly the same, you fade into the scenery. Looking at my blonde hair, Gad remarked, "I like surfer hair streaked with a few broad strokes of sunshine." Even if you bleach your hair, keep the contrasts—a darker shade underneath and a few large, light streaks on top.

His individually mixed hair-color preparations often contain at least three shades of one or more color families. That adds subtlety and depth to highlights. He adds colors gradually as he needs them for different parts of the head. For example, he might mix medium brown and light ash blonde as a base then add a few drops of titian red for warm highlights on top. The darker base color underneath gives hair depth and richness. Highlights give hair energy and bounce. Based on his approach, you might divide your hair into three sections:

- Bottom: from the ear lobe to the neck
- Middle: from the ear lobe to the top of the ear across the back of the head
- Top: in front of the ear to the top of the head and to the face

For a sun-kissed look, use the darkest color on bottom, a lighter shade in the middle, and the lightest on top. You can blend some of all three like a painter. Whether you use permanent hair color on the roots or a less damaging temporary rinse, choose colors that best suit your complexion without makeup.

Discover Your Style

Gad has developed a style sense based on years of experience with people who have great taste, including fashion editors, designers, photographers, and top fashion models. He advises neophytes to develop their unique style by watching old movies, scouring magazines, reading books, and attending art shows and museums. "Tear out pictures of clothes, hair, and makeup styles from magazines, but also flowers, gardens, beautiful homes, and people. Put them into a scrap book. Eventually you will use your impressions to forge your own style."

When I ask Gad specific style questions, his favorite answer is: "It depends." His approach is based on your appearance and lifestyle. "A person should have a number of different styles depending on her life situation, her work, and activities. Style is not about fashion. Style is knowing exactly the right thing to wear for the occasion." He said, "To have personal style, to find yourself, you have to find things that look good on *you,* things that enhance *your* body." For a lot of us, that means slimming.

Dressing to Slim

Gad uses design for slimming. A turtleneck slims and lengthens the neck. A tight-fitting T-shirt or sweater worn *outside* a flared skirt or pants slims and lengthens the waist. But sticking the shirt into a wide belt shortens the waist and cuts a slimming line in half. Clothes designed with an empire shape balance an overly large figure. "Nicely fitted jackets that are snug at the shoulder and bust but not too tight at the waist are also good. Nothing should fit too tightly on a large figure." In general, clothes should graze over the body and not be too loose or too tight. For a short torso, pants that are cut low at the waist lengthen better than a high-cut or thick waistband. Pants with a tight waist make the hips balloon. A tight-waisted skirt is slimming, but not pants. For beautiful suits, he recommends Jill Saunders, Prada, Mark Jacobs, and especially Yves St. Laurent. *Bien sur.*

For people who are short and square, single-breasted suits elongate more than double-breasted. Gad advises to deemphasize the middle by avoiding baggy or very straight-cut jackets. They should fall not too far or close to the body. Avoid huge shoulder pads, but a slight increase in shoulder width slims the waist. Dark matte colors such as black, navy, and charcoal reduce bulk. If you wear a tweed or plaid jacket, wear a solid color shirt or vest underneath. Pin stripes and Prince of Wales fabrics make good suits for slimming.

Men can look taller with polished-looking hair and an inner shoe lift. If your legs are longer than your torso, wear pants that are low-waisted. If you have more torso than leg, wear higher-waisted pants. If you have a large torso and wide shoulders, you can wear a shirt outside of the pants to deemphasize the waist.

Job Interviews, Auditions, and Style

Gad advises people to prepare for an interview like a performer. "You need to mentally create the physicalities of the job—how you need to look in that setting. You are taking on a character. Think about the job description. If it is corporate, look polished. Look as though you can get your act together and have everything under control. Your hair should be smooth, not fuzzy and wild.

Pull long hair back in a ponytail. A fabulous suit and great shoes all work together. You may want a skirt that's a little sexy, but make it sexy and powerful."

A television anchorwoman has to be more polished, tailored, and professional-looking than an actress. He has worked with Heather Locklear, Jacqueline Smith, and Paula Zahn. "For television," he says, "you want the proportions of the body and head to look balanced. You can't be all hair or shoulders. Colors can't be too bright. If you wear blue, add slimming black pants or skirt. Also slimming are a black outfit with a blue blazer for a dash of color on top. Black gives you a good silhouette. Put on a black suit first, then throw on a touch of blue just to make everything pop."

For auditions, Gad suggests, "Go dressed like the character. Casting people want to see something of the character they are looking for without your having to stretch." Eileen Heckart, the famous stage and screen actress, told me she always prepared for parts by studying the period when the character lived. Books from that time tell you how people thought, moved, and spoke then, also the activities that would have shaped their style identity. For example, Victorian women were trussed up in tight corsets that limited movement and breathing, therefore energy.

Jewelry—How Much?

Gad finds jewelry very aging. "Older women wear a lot. It weighs them down! If you have nice jewelry, before you go out the door, always take one thing off. If you wear rings, earrings, necklace, and a bracelet, it's far too much! If you wear something low cut and your chest and shoulders are nude and your hair is up, you may want to wear a little piece around your neck so you don't look bare. It is all balance."

As you will see, Clif deRaita, Georgette Klinger's National Director of Makeup, recommends the color of certain gems to enhance a corresponding complexion. It is not surprising that traditional Asian doctors consider the *energy* of metals and gems to have healing qualities. Silver is considered cooling and gold warming. We can adapt their theories to jewelry. If you want to cool hot emotions or fever or if the weather is hot, wear something cool and lightweight like diamonds, crystal, silver, or white gold. If you want to spark energy and warmth, wear gold, coral, or amber. If you need moisture try wearing pearls while drinking American ginseng tea. If you are feeling anxious or hyperactive, wear a heavyweight beaded necklace to anchor you. Consider how the weight, color, and vibrational quality of jewelry affects your energy.

Model Tricks for Reversing Imperfections

Even models don't look perfect first thing in the morning. Here are some of their tricks to look good in photos. You can give yourself a facelift without plastic surgery using a clear tape available at beauty supply companies. Place the tape along your facial hairline and at the jaw line near the front of the neck. Then use special elastic bands that pull back the entire face and attach in your hair. Cover the tape with your hair or a wig. Or tightly braid your hair into a pony tail at the top and attach a heavy weight, which draws your hair (and face) back.

When fatigue gives complexion a dull, ashen, or dry appearance, you can swallow 1 tablespoon of olive oil daily. Flaxseed oil capsules reduce cholesterol; the vitamin A in olive oil is beautifying for hair and skin. Another holistic trick is homeopathic silver (argentum nitricum) which helps the skin to retain freshness. Depending on the dilution, the remedy reduces dryness originating from deep inside, from stressed internal organs to the skin's surface. Homeopathic argentum nitricum 200C, a minute trace, is recommended for long-term burnout, insomnia, and impulsiveness. Take one dose at bedtime. Less dilute argentum nitricum 30C is recommended for acute dry skin, crinkly lines, skin cracks, blood shot eyes, and feeling overheated. Take a dose as needed between meals.

Clothing Colors vs. Black and White

Gad and the other stylists I interviewed choose clothing colors that complement skin and hair color. For example, Gad advises ruddy complexions to wear muted green shades. Like a painter, he knows that paired primary colors strongly affect each other. Pale shades mute each other; bright shades emphasize line. For example, pale green cools red, but bright red and green juxtaposed make each other jump in contrast. If you want to deemphasize your waistline, don't wear a red shirt next to green pants. You can balance a color choice with a scarf. Says Gad, "Choose a scarf color that is flattering and wear it around your face so that your complexion benefits from its reflection."

Gad, who often wears black, feels that "Color makes us look younger. However, there are good uses for white and black." He likes white for a business look. "Wear a crisp cotton shirt with a suit. It brightens skin, reduces wrinkles, and makes you look softer." I have wondered why so many people wear black in New York. It seems funereal or pseudo-Victorian. Gad told me, "You have to feel very successful and strong when you wear black. It does not lighten or brighten the skin as white does, but it creates a kind of mystique. It is a chic color that is extremely slimming."

Color According to a Hair Genius

Hair color is a major factor in determining clothing colors, according to Gad. Hair and complexion colors are the top of the pyramid for most stylists. From there, you can determine clothing colors and shapes. Here is chart to summarize what Gad told me:

Hair Color	Most Flattering Clothing Colors
Red	Green, pink, black, and blue
Blonde	Black, red, teal blue, or cobalt blue with brown accents, taupe, grays, and olive green
Brunette	Orange, pink, and yellow
Black	Bold colors and shiny, day glo finishes

Gad, who insists on cutting hair during the full moon, prefers warmer, darker hair shades during winter and lighter shades for summer. But the choice depends on you, the moon, and that special magic that makes style.

Clif deRaita: A Holistic Approach

Another way to look at color is Clif deRaita's use of seasonal colors according to your natural complexion and hair color. His advice most resembles a holistic, energetic approach because he uses colors and jewelry to bring out the complexion's potential beauty. Here is a chart to summarize what he told me:

Natural Coloring	Recommended Clothing and Jewelry
Ash blondes and towheads	"Summer colors": ice pastels and driftwood Jewelry: cooling silver and diamonds
Warm, strawberry, and golden blondes	"Spring colors": grass green, daffodil yellow, peach, off white, beige, and tan Jewelry: coral, turquoise, and gold
Redheads or brunettes with pink skin and blue or green eyes	"Autumn colors": orange, gold, ochre, burnt umber, Indian coral, paprika, orange-red, pimiento, bright purple, greens, and blues, especially turquoise; add green or brown accents to black
Brunettes or black hair with sallow, olive and darker complexions; Asian- and African-American people	Intense colors to the max: royal blue, true red, deep purple, white, black, emerald green (pastel clothing for summer) Jewelry: silver, diamonds, and platinum

Clif finds gold too yellow for darker complexions because, "it brings out the unflattering yellow or sallow undertones of the skin." He believes that a person can make any colored outfit work by coordinating the makeup palette accordingly. Lipstick is especially important. His golden rule is: "Complement Mother Nature's handiwork. She knows what she is doing."

You Be the Judge

Try on Gad's and Clif's color recommendations. First, use your natural hair and complexion colors as a guide. Place pieces of colored paper or cloth against your face. Observe them in sunlight and artificial light. See the difference they make for your skin, hair, and style. Then try other colors with wigs and makeup. What fabrics look the best with them? What do they do for your energy and mood? What or who do they remind you of? What look do you want to create?

A group of close women friends I know get together periodically to offer each other their favorite used clothing. It's nice to see something that has special meaning—your Dad's shirt or your maternity dress—worn by someone you like. It might lead to style discoveries.

Marietta Carter-Narcisse: From the Ground Up

If you want to study makeup with a beauty pro, this highly successful Los Angeles professional makeup artist shares her knowledge in one-week intensive workshops she calls Boot Camp. Based on her wide experience in film, the class covers everything you need to know to work in the industry. Marietta, originally from Barbados, has a cosmetology and aesthetics license as well as a Bachelor's Degree in Chemistry and Psychology. She told me, "I dropped out of med school to turn my hobby into a lucrative career."

Boot Camp covers résumé preparation, interview techniques, and deal negotiations along with makeup for film, television, print, and salon. You learn basic skin care as well as basic color and lighting theory, how to determine undertones, product knowledge and blending techniques, men's grooming, and makeup trends. She is well suited to teach professional makeup artists. Marietta has worked as image consultant for Natalie Cole and Whoopi Goldberg, and has many film credits, including *The Red Violin, Sphere, Eve's Bayou, The Long Kiss Goodnight,* and *Malcolm X.* She has worked with stars including Samuel L. Jackson, Michelle Pfeiffer, Debbie Morgan, Cindy Crawford, Angela Bassett, Ellen Barkin, Diahann Carroll, Lynn Whitfield, Woody Harrelson, and Denzel Washington.

Makeup and Dark Complexions

I asked Marietta if there were any special makeup issues presented by darker complexions. She said that the texture of the skin dictates the consistency of the foundation used—whether cream, powder, liquid, or other. Mature skin requires moisture. You have to use a richer moisturizer and more oil in the foundation. She explained how she mixed makeup foundation colors based on the prominent undertones in the skin. Covering extra pigmentation, flaws, or tattoos is done with an undercoat of orange. Finally, she said simply: "Skin is skin. I treat it all the same. Actors need to take care of their health to take care of their skin." No matter if you start from inside or outside, health is beauty and beauty health.

Makeup and Lighting for a Youthful Look on Screen

Television makeup requires heavy application that covers everything, unlike film, where complexion flaws show. The most flattering television makeup I ever had was sprayed on with a blow gun that evens out lines and blemishes. Unless you are the star, you may have to do your own makeup for television appearances. It pays to know some basics.

- Use matte makeup. Television lights make skin shine and look oily.
- Avoid glitter or day-glo makeup colors, except for lip gloss.
- Avoid prints, tweeds, and plaids: they make the camera eye jump.

On screen and in print, we are at the mercy of the lighting crew. White light drains facial color and can make you look tired. Warm or slightly gold lights are flattering for most people. A gauze screen placed over a light or a camera lens can cut years of age. An indirect light shining up to your face from waist level fills in wrinkles. An overhead spot light elongates features. You can't always have a talk with the lighting crew or move as you want to on set, but be aware of where the camera and lighting are. If you are choosing an outfit for a demo tape that will be copied many times, be aware that red colors "bleed." Red looks smeared in copies.

Photography, like television, requires heavier makeup because of bright lighting. Before you have professional photographs done, have a professional makeup consultation. It might involve a change in hair color that you will have to get used to.

The Calypso Queen

Recently, Marietta has crossed over from applying makeup to manufacturing an exciting beauty line called Calypso Cosmetics. Marietta has vivid childhood memories of her mom combining different types of leaves that she had picked from trees and vines in the yard. There were olive bush, sugar apple and pear leaf, sweet aloe, ginger root, dried orange peel, and others. She steeped these concoctions to make "Bush Tea that cured everything from a runny nose to a tummy ache." Marietta has remained fascinated with herbs, flowers, and spices. Calypso Cosmetics uses the same island fragrances that tantalized her senses as a child. Marietta has reason to be proud when she says,

"Calypso Cosmetics marry my love of the fashion and beauty industry with my love of chemistry and the natural healing property of what our earth has to offer. Additionally, I want to share the history of a people, one that is rich with tenacity, perseverance, color, and loads of a 'soon cum' (sooner or later). My people are easy come easy go, typically living a laid-back lifestyle. The best way I know how to share this rich culture is through my love of what I know best: cosmetics."

Her products are named after a region, flower, food, or colloquial expression taken from the unique lifestyle of Barbados, encompassing African, French, Dutch, Spanish, and English influences. "My grandfather, at the ripe young age of 101, still massages his skin with a concoction of plants, olive and coconut oils, to maintain the moisture in his skin and keep his youthful glow. He'll also sip a shot or two of rum daily."

For a trip to the islands without leaving home, take a Bajan Bush Bath, soak in some Anguilla Bath Salts or Lait De Bain (milk bath). Lather up with Savon De Corps (handmade body soaps) or exfoliate with Bequia Body Scrub. Shampoo with "Ganga" Marietta's Rasta Shampoo Bar then immerse hair in Rasta Hair Oil. For massage or for dry skin and hair, there is The Standpipe Body Oil and Tropical Body Butter. One delicious body butter is called Mango Chutney! With the stretch of your imagination and some island music, you will be limbo dancing in the tub.

Anguilla Bath Salts are named after the island in the Eastern Caribbean. They blend pure Dead Sea mineral salts, Epsom salts, baking soda, exotic nut oils, citric acid, and pure essential and/or fragrance oils. Selections include Anthurium Lily, which is great for dry skin; Boston Beach (my favorite), a spicy mixture of juniper berry, gardenia, and bay; Creole Lady, made with roses; Papiamento, for those who love lavender; Plumeria; and Sweet Lime, a hypnotic island scent of lemon verbena, lime, and calendula.

I also love Marietta's Bajan Bush Bath teas bags you steep in the tub. Their names and ingredients are fun. For example, Nelson Street is named after the old red-light district of Barbados. It's a sexy blend of lavender, rosemary, thyme, and jasmine with essential oils. Calypso Cosmetics also include Dominican Lip Balm in delicious flavors like Honey Lemonade and Lime Squash. They are made with shea, mango, and cocoa butters; beeswax; coconut and sweet almond oils; along with essential oils.

Going Native: Body Piercing and Tattoos

Do you have ear or body piercing or tattoos? You probably never thought about the acupuncture meridians located there. My pierced nose eventually became a hassle. If you pierce an acupuncture point (there are hundreds) it can cause internal reactions. I had punctured a large intestine point, which infected when I ate spicy food. The ear contains acupuncture points for internal organs, the spine, the nervous system, the head, and limbs—basically the entire body. The head points are in the ear lobe and the spine is along the inner ridge of the ear. Acupuncture treatments for stopping addictions, nervous anxiety, and weight loss work quite well with ear points. Consider having an acupuncturist mark the best points to be pierced before having it done in a shop.

Tattoos are common. In China, women tattoo their eyelids and eyebrows. The dye penetrates the skin and is hard to remove if you change your mind. Be very careful to guide your tattoo artist for the look you want. Remember that your face will change as you age. You don't want a frozen-faced look. See the eye chapter in this book when drawing the perfect eyebrow.

Stick-on, removable body tattoos are safer and less painful than permanent ones. If you choose to have it done permanently, herbal antibiotic pills such as oldenlandia (bai hua sheshecao) or andrographis (chuan xin lian) taken with acne cures such as Lien Chiao Pai Tu Pien will reduce inflammation discomfort. Yunnan Paiyao increases circulation and speeds healing of punctures. Herbal alternatives include goldenseal and dandelion as anti-inflammatory herbs and homeopathic arnica montana 30C to reduce bruising and swelling.

Especially for Men

Marietta Carter-Narcisse prefers a look for men she calls clean and simple. "I usually clean the beard and moustache up with a clipper with a guard on it. I like it close to the skin, very neat. If hairs are missing I usually fill in with a pencil close to the color of the hair so that everything is full and natural. Men should be style conscious. They should realize that their skin is part of them and they should treat it accordingly. If men have oily skin, they should wash their faces morning, noon, and night and use oil-free moisturizers as well as oil-blotting tissues throughout the day. Cosmetics are not meant for women only. It's not feminine."

Lola's Way

Lee Strasberg, creator-director of the Actors Studio, once said about Marilyn Monroe, "I saw that what she looked like was not what she really was, and what was going on inside her was not what was going on outside, and that always means there may be something to work with." Using inner life experience is the essence of Method Acting: we look inward and outward at the same time. Montgomery Clift, Marilyn's co-star in *The Misfits*, said: "She listens, wants, cares. Every pore of that lovely translucent skin is alive, open every moment—even though this world could make her vulnerable to being hurt . . . I would rather work with her than any other actress. I adore her." Marilyn, who loved the camera, shared her narcissism generously with us. We can't take our eyes off her. She created herself in front of her mirror during several hours of makeup before each performance. Makeup is much more than coverup. It uncovers. It can reveal your secret self.

The final word comes from Michael Foster, novelist and biographer of heroic women, including Adah Isaacs Menken, the first American superstar sex goddess. Born impoverished, Jewish, and part black, she created the death-defying stage role for Byron's Mazeppa. Michael defines style as "personal expression." He says, "Without that, style is only foppery. The energy, vivacity, and scope of great people are attractive because they have courage to be themselves."

The Five Elements of Beauty

So far in this book we have observed your body, complexion, hair, walk, and fragrance. Although your vitality and looks vary with life's events, you are born with an energetic, physical, and personality type that suggests the Five Elements: Fire, Earth, Metal, Water, and Wood. Eventually, you will be able to observe their effects for yourself and others. Just for fun, intuit your Element type by looking over the following descriptions. It is not a quiz. Your Element(s) has strengths and weaknesses, advantages and disadvantages, just like your appearance and personality. Which celebrities or Elements seem most like yourself or friends? How have they profited from their Element? How might your Element(s) enhance your beauty?

Fire, Earth, Metal, Water, and Wood Celebrities

Fire

Fire is warm, emotional, or flashy. Fire people like to act, sing, and emote. They can be fiery or cold as ice as the occasion suits them. They are often slender, delicate, graceful, and elegant. They have shapely hands and fingernails. When feeling hot, romantic, and emotional, their hands are warm and red. Fire celebrities include Nicole Kidman, Gwyneth Paltrow, Michelle Pfeiffer, and Halle Berry. The great Greta Garbo (a Metal type) played a Fire type in the movie *Camille,* where the tragic heroine (Margarite) describes herself as, "nervous, sick, sad, or too gay." The Baron says of her, "So much heart and so little sense."

Earth

Earth is generous to a fault, works hard, and worries about detail. A hearty laugh or quick joke is a sign of a happy Earth person. They can be peace-makers and self-sacrificing parents. Catherine Zeta-Jones has said, "I was born to breed." The world needs more stunning Earth types like her. Daisy Fuentes looks like an Earth type—sweet as cinnamon. A healthy Earth type wants to make everyone comfortable. They love cooking, family, home, and music. Earth requires stability and roots. A sick Earth type, or someone suffering an Earth-related problem such as divorce or a job change, can be demanding and depressed. Digestive herbs will help anyone deal with major change.

Metal

Metal can be dedicated, single-minded, or reclusive. Metal people often enjoy working alone or drive themselves hard with stimulants and addictions. When fatigued, they become weak and breathless. They are tall, slim supermodels, and everyone admires their cool manner and dignified walk—Tyra Banks, Katouche, Naomi Campbell, Karen Alexander, Shakara, and Beverly Johnson. Unless tweaked by plastic surgery, they often have a prominent nose as a distinctive facial feature. Their facial structure and habits can give them a nasal or breathy voice. Metal celebrities include Penelope Cruz, Sarah Jessica Parker, Donatella Versace, Michelle Williams, Adrien Brody, and Ralph Fiennes.

Metal can easily be intensely sexy and sensitive. We want to see what is behind the attractive shell. Actor John Cusack displays a Metal type prerogative by being a loner. Metal's sex appeal is focus and intensity—you hope that your Metal lover is dreamy over, going nuts, or pouting about only you.

Water

Water types have to fight excess weight. They have drive, courage, and stamina when healthy. One splendid example is Elizabeth Taylor who has become an ocean of compassion. Isabella Rossellini also has lovely facial features that suggest the Water Element. Her makeup line, Manifesto, stresses individuality. As she sees it, "Beauty standards in contemporary culture are geared toward blonde, blue-eyed women in their 20s—and should be ignored. You can't win if you go down that route. And I like to win." That kind of determination highlights the Water Element.

Water can be an audacious, in-your-face, break-the-rules type like Roseanne or a vamp like Lana Turner. Great examples of the sexual heat generated by Water and Metal combined are Marilyn Monroe and Jennifer Lopez.

Water's drive and Metal's vision can also produce crusaders for justice or business tycoons, like Oprah Winfrey.

Wood

Male Wood types are tough, hard driving, muscle bound, and hungry. They have square regular features and athletic bodies. Handsome examples are Ben Affleck, Daniel Day Lewis, Jeremy Irons, Clint Eastwood, Brad Pitt, Michael Douglas, Harrison Ford, Russell Crowe, and George Clooney. Women with balanced Wood facial features are not bad either—Cameron Diaz, Brooke Shields, and Amanda Peet. They have strong athletic bodies that enjoy movement. Sick Wood types have spasm pain from headaches, as well as allergies and hot tempers. They make snap decisions about people and scripts.

Otherwise, to find a Wood type, listen to the voice. The Wood voice has clarity, crisp consonants, and clipped vowels. It is neither sing-songish like Earth nor sighing like Metal. A tight jaw can signal Wood's determination. Katharine Hepburn's forthright, optimistic character is a great example of the enlightened determination and insight of Wood and Metal.

The Five Elements encompass every aspect of health, beauty, and well-being. The following chapter engages your most subtle aspect of beauty and seduction—your voice.

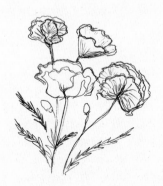

16

Your Voice Tells a Story

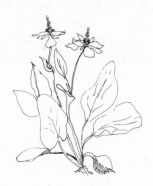

"Joy rests on truth and strength in the heart
and is expressed by gentleness to others."
—*THE I CHING OR BOOK OF CHANGES*
(Richard Wilhelm, translator)

Your voice creates a mental image of you. That sort of synergy has been expressed well by Laura Linney, who starred with Jim Carrey in Paramount Pictures' *The Truman Show* in 1998: "When what you hear and what you see and what you taste are all combined—that's pretty damn sexy."

What image do you want to create? Cool, elegant, moody, tough, and/or sexy? To make an impression at a meeting or audition, you might study examples such as actors or celebrities. "If you want to cultivate your voice and breath," I was told by an vocal coach, "listen to the violin. Good musical phrasing and correct breathing are as smooth as a violin."

Felix Mendelssohn's elegant violin concerto in E minor sums up the musical language of the nineteenth century. Mendelssohn, slender and pale with dark, sensitive features, resembled his friend Chopin. They created an emaciated Romantic look that later shaped James Dean and Frank Sinatra. Their thin, intense look has morphed into today's heroin chic. Mendelssohn and Chopin were examples of the Metal Element's sunken-cheek pallor. They died young from disappointment. Felix died soon after his sister Fanny, who had been his constant companion. It was as though Narcissus could not face look-ing into the pool without seeing his female self. The downside of the Metal Element is depression, addiction, and asthma. Is that the energy you want your voice to express?

Use Chinese energetic principles in this chapter and create the *sound* you want. The voice penetrates deeply and makes a lasting impression. Billie Hol-iday, Judy Garland, and Hank Williams became celebrities and sex symbols without being great beauties. We loved their *voices.* This chapter covers the energetic basis of a strong, clear voice, which may be used however you pre-fer. The voice can be a sword to defeat an enemy or an elixir of love. Your voice can be used in performance to create a character. You need not have one voice for all occasions; adaptability is the essence of beauty and good acting.

Inhale Deeply and Relax Completely

A flexible speaking and singing voice is built on breath support. Its resonance comes from the overtones of freely circulating sound. Traditional Chinese doctors turn vocal culture into diagnosis. They believe that a pleasing voice is one sign of a strong heart and balanced emotions. They observe unusual or strained vocal tone as a sign of imbalance in the Five Elements. The vocal techniques that I share will connect you with the reservoir of feelings, colors, memories, and music that you carry inside.

A relaxed voice is pleasing because you sense that the speaker or singer is comfortable. We cringe when hearing a harsh voice because our muscles tense in sympathy. A shrill voice is unsettling or frightening. Over time, a rough voice can become an unfortunate part of one's identity. Many people are insensitive to the unsettling effect their voice may have on others. Imag-ine a love song sung with a sand paper snarl or a groan. It is important to be able to hear and project the voice (and personality) that you want.

To help you to recognize your vocal quality, I have included diagnostic information gleaned from the Chinese Five Elements: Fire, Earth, Metal, Water, and Wood. When you can recognize yourself vocally and improve technique, you will be able to match the persona you want with the sound you make.

Your Voice and The Five Elements

Vocal quality, strength, and habits indicate the vitality of the Five Elements. You can tell a lot about someone by listening to their voice. With training, you can *hear* where their feelings are coming from or which Element is engaged. Do they giggle, hum or singsong, pant for breath, groan words, or spit con-sonants? Each Element has a contented balanced sound as well as a sound of alarm or weakness.

In Chapter 8, we applied the Five Elements to personal fragrance. In the following section, I describe vocal problems associated with each Element. I tend to describe vocal *problems* because I am a health practitioner, but each voice has its charm and advantages. Daily habits and temporary emotions always affect the voice.

For example, you may be an affable Earth person who loves congenial people and sweet foods but, because of stress and fatigue, your voice can take on a shrill urgency signaling trouble in the Fire Element. The exercises, teas, and other recommendations found in this chapter can help your voice to regain its naturally healthy sound. On the other hand, you may be required to develop a stage or screen character who embodies emotions boiling over. Using that character's (that Element's) voice and gestures will take you into their body and soul.

The following chart shows examples of the voice, the associated Element, the location of possible physical discomforts, and emotions possibly expressed. What does your voice sound like?

Voice	Element	Physical Discomforts	Emotions
Chatter, giggle, shriek, stutter	Fire	Heart and chest	Joy or anxiety
Singsong, whine	Earth	Digestive area Hypoglycemia	Relaxed, romantic Worry
Breathless	Metal	Lungs, fatigue	Depression
Groan	Water	Backache, fatigue	Apathy, fear
Yelling, tight jaw, staccato	Wood	Head, chest muscles	Urgency, anger, frustration, emphatic
Shaking	Wood	Nervous insomnia, weakness	Nervousness

Fire

The Fire Element helps regulate physical and emotional temperature. When imbalanced, the Fire person boils over with high emotions. They can be anxious and highly expressive. People who talk constantly show Fire's imbalance. When overstimulated, they chatter aimlessly in order to hear themselves, and their laugh is a shriek. They may stutter. Caffeine or stimulants, which Fire types tend to abuse, make them anxious, insomniac, and relentless. A Fire person may be a visionary or hysteric—but is never boring. They are frequently sentimental and are all heart. In fact, their heart can be troubled by irregularities, murmurs, and plaque.

The Fire Voice—Overcome Anxiety

Since the Fire Element is influenced by heart function, a voice that is moderated, smooth, and evenly pitched indicates health. A tone that is shrill, high-pinched, strained, shrieking, squealing, or "down in the dumps" indicates a problem with vital energy and circulation. The more high-pitched the chatter or squeal, the more stressed are the emotions. Anxiety is fast and hot. A stutter is a sign of emotional arrhythmia, when the heart feels off center. Vivien Leigh playing Blanche DuBois in *A Streetcar Named Desire* used the full range of emotions expressed by her voice. Traditional Chinese medicine believes that a troubled Fire Element can slip into madness. When a heart is broken, imbalance quickly follows.

Teas to soothe a shrill voice are heavy in nature, such as bay leaf. Ginger, mint, and licorice tea can sometimes help the Fire person to feel more grounded. Add a twist of lemon peel for flavor. One-quarter teaspoon of Siberian ginseng powder added to a cup of hot water makes a soothing relaxing tea.

Caffeine, insomnia, and cold weather can make any voice grind to a spasm. Warm rosebud tea opens the chest, freeing circulation for enhanced comfort.

Earth

The Earth person may be round in the middle from eating sweets, their favorite foods, or thin from chronic indigestion and diarrhea. Healthy Earth people are good natured. Their center (bread basket) is the secure platform for their emotions, familial involvements (often complicated), and lifestyle. They enjoy the comforts of home, good cooking, and congenial friends. Some develop hypoglycemia followed by diabetes. They require extra zinc and exercise to help balance their blood sugar.

If troubled by unstable loving relationships, frequent moving, or job changes; if they do not feel appreciated; or if they eat and drink the wrong things; they can become depressed or sick. They seek stability, commitment, and affection and can generously reciprocate.

The Earth Voice—Overcome Digestive Weakness

A lot of classical music singers are Earth people. They love pasta. The Earth Element, according to Chinese medicine, is associated with the sweet flavor and the singing sound. When the Earth person feels off-center, they sound off-center. It's hard to tell exactly where the voice is coming from. It's not supported by breath and sounds as though it is not connected to the body. It wobbles and fades off pitch. It can dip and bob in a twang or sound sweet but lack resonance. The Earth person whines depending on how rooted they feel.

Hyper- or hypothyroid conditions may develop in extreme cases, leading to exhibitionism (often singing) or catatonic withdrawal.

The Earth voice can be a beautiful singing voice when supported with steady breath that comes from deep down. Standing straight helps vocal production because you feel rooted. Unfortunately, most of the time we have to speak while moving. To feel more grounded and build your basis of breath support, massage your feet daily. Then do this simple stretch that yogis call the cat: on all fours, with knees and fists to the floor, bend the spine to make it first concave then convex. Dip the spine down toward the floor then raise it toward the ceiling. Follow the easy, slow movement of your spine with your head and eyes. This bends you in the middle for greater flexibility.

To help free your middle, stand with arms straight at your sides. Turn up the palms to the ceiling. Lift the arms to shoulder height and twist only the trunk, not the hips, slowly from side to side. Inhale as you face ahead and exhale as you twist.

The herbs that help you to sing, speak, and think clearly eliminate mucus congestion. Mucus is increased by sweets, dairy products, and beer; inadequate exercise; too much sleep; humid weather; and emotional upset. Barley soup reduces phlegm. A tea made with fennel seeds, ginger, lemongrass, and mint will brighten your voice. Add a dash of cardamom to lift energy and mood. If you have diabetes, avoid all sweets except up to ¼ teaspoon of cinnamon daily. It is recommended to help balance blood sugar.

Homeopathic remedies useful for chronic mucus congestion include two forms of potassium: homeopathic kali. mur. 6x and homeopathic kali. sulph. 6x. You might add one dose of each to a quart of water and sip it throughout the day.

Metal

The Metal Element affects breathing and the elimination of toxins. The Metal Element represents the energy system comprised of the lung, large intestine, and skin. The nose can be prominent like a bulb or beak.

Metal people can be wan and breathless when tired. They are prone to upper-respiratory-tract or sinus infections, mucus congestion, asthma, skin blemishes, and eczema. They can become addicted to dangerous substances, including cigarettes and drugs, when they live behind a smokescreen. Since breathing can be a survival issue for them, they might hide from people to avoid talking. They might develop a ghostly pallor or chronic cough unless they energize their breathing. More than a few actors and singers I know have told me that if it were not for singing, their asthma would have killed them.

Metal people tend to be loners among the Five Elements. They enjoy solitary, spiritual, or artistic work that stretches their imagination and talent.

The Metal Voice—Learn How to Breathe

The Metal voice can be nasal or hoarse from mucus and inflammation. A husky sound or dry cough also indicates chronic thirst, fever, or a cold. If energy is low (or when imitating Marilyn Monroe), the voice is breathy. Marilyn was a combination of Water and Metal Elements—at best a gifted actress who loved approbation, and at worst a lonely, frightened girl.

Metal people develop a weepy sound when they are tired. To build breath support and increase oxygen, reduce dairy products and sweets in your diet. Add antimucus apples, carrots, and radishes. If you have chronic thirst, drink American ginseng tea. Exercise in order to perspire, which helps reduce mucus congestion and fat. Lift weights to build strong shoulder and upper back muscles. Do it by placing weights at shoulder height and lifting upward in order to stretch your neck. Do squats and walk daily to firm the legs. The visualizations and exercises that follow in this chapter will help to deepen your breath.

Sinus Congestion, Allergies, and Shortness of Breath

One way to recognize trouble in the Metal Element is to hear a nasal voice, mucus congestion, or shortness of breath. Singers, speakers, and media personalities especially need remedies to clear sinus passages, throat, and lungs without mind-dulling or skin-drying side effects. A pleasant everyday Chinese instant beverage made by Yin/Yang Sisters is called Breathe Free. Large quantities of the boxes containing individually foil-wrapped concentrated herbal powder have been sold to New Yorkers since September 11, 2001. You just add water and drink it hot or cold to facilitate breathing, clear allergic and stress mucus congestion, and refresh the lungs. Its healing herbs include skullcap, ligustrum, angelica, siler, black dates, notopterygum root, magnolia flower, and xanthium fruit. (See more about the Yin/Yang Sisters brand in Chapter 17, Survival Skills.)

If you are troubled by phlegm and sad feelings, which often go together, I recommend homeopathic pulsatilla 30C. It reduces chest tightness and enhances breathing. The remedy makes you feel like you are standing on a mountain, watching the sunrise and feeling clear, cheerful, and content.

Do not overuse the herb echinacea during flu season. No matter what you may hear about its wonderful effects from health authorities, echinacea is extremely drying. Its use is recommend only during the first day or two of an upper-respiratory-tract infection. After that, it can aggravate sweating to the point of a sore throat and dizziness.

To moisten the throat and prevent irritation, take the advice of Shirley Varret. She told me that before walking on stage to sing an opera, she takes a dose of homeopathic calc. sulph. 6x, a cleanser that boosts immunity. All the above remedies for reducing mucus apply to both Earth and Metal people.

Water

The Water Element is a primary source of our energy and immunity. A tired Water person tends to stagnate and feel overcome by problems. If hormone imbalances develop from illness or fatigue, there may be extra facial hair. If the person is weak or has a tiring lifestyle, a variety of energy, immunity, and sexuality complaints will likely result.

For most of us, a wise balance of energy, drive, and rest is required to prevent burnout. However, sick and driven Water Element people find it hard to add 1 and 1 and get 2: they think they can abuse their energy, consume whatever they wish, travel anywhere any time, work until all hours, and get away with it. Some highly intellectual people completely lose touch with their body. Others drive themselves hard enough to feel the pain. They may believe in magic or fall into bottomless pits of exhaustion and apathy.

At best, the Water person is heroic and courageous—a pathfinder. At worst, Water becomes paranoid (hyperadrenal), while looking for problems before they occur. An exemplary Metal/Water person is Andy Warhol. If you can find pictures of him before his plastic surgery, his prominent Metal nose is apparent.

The Water Voice—Prevent Exhaustion and Fear

Since adrenal energy is so important for the Water Element as well as for speaking and singing, Water types need to take special precautions in order to protect their vitality and endurance. Otherwise, the voice will develop its characteristic exhausted, groaning quality. Fatigue makes it harder to remain on pitch. Vocal stress occurs when breath cannot support the voice and the speaker or singer clenches the throat to push out a sound. Backache and shortness of breath also complicate vocal problems.

To increase endurance, add a combination of several ginsengs to your daily health routine. The ginseng family of herbs are adaptogens because they help us to adapt to stress. They reduce fatigue and temperature sensitivity (see Chapter 3).

The following methods relax the lower back and facilitate deep inhalation. To support vitality, gently massage inward toward the navel from 2 inches away on either side of the navel. Also massage the soles of the feet and the toes in order to relax circulation in the legs and lower back. Lie on the floor with a wooden roller pressing against the kidney area, which is on your back opposite the navel.

Wood

The Wood Element controls muscles, tendons, joints, movement, creativity, and vision. The healthy, happy Wood person is a traveler, dancer, athlete, or someone who moves first and fast in new directions. Their body tends to be angular and often stiff. They need exercise and room to breathe. In the spring, or any time they abuse their energy, they can be plagued with allergies, aches, PMS, temper tantrums, or insomnia.

Wood people need to develop wisdom and generosity. Like a young ram, they accept few limits for themselves or others. Their perfectionism can give them migraines or stage fright. Given a clear field or hard-won patience, they can and do move mountains.

The Wood Voice—Prevent Spasms and Aches

The Wood person can have a tight, determined jaw. Their consonants are staccato. Their normal voice can sound pinched like yelling. Breath support can be weak if muscles are too tight. They need to gently bend, swim, do yoga, soak in an Epsom salts bath, or take a nap to relax before a performance. Homeopathic magnesium (mag. phos. 6x) taken several times daily can help them to avoid spasms, stuttering, and muscle pain. Cleansing herbs such as dandelion and honeysuckle tea can help prevent excess acid conditions.

Basic Breathing Exercise for All Types

To calm the voice and build breath, I recommend the following exercise for all vocal types. It works especially well for anyone who lives under stress and overuses stimulants such as chocolate and caffeine drinks.

- Lie flat and place your palms on to your lower abdomen below the navel.
- Relax the head, neck, and chest completely.
- Inhale deeply and slowly into the lower abdomen.
- Relax your lower back to the floor.
- As you exhale downward toward your feet, imagine an ocean wave.
- Let yourself melt. Put troubles aside for another day.
- Continue breathing deeply, while relaxing the face for several minutes.

Some people like to place a weight such as the yellow pages onto the abdomen in order to increase muscle strength. If you choose to do so, avoid tensing muscles anywhere. Relax completely and imagine that your abdomen is a beehive full of happy worker bees. You are the queen enjoying your home. Let the breath be a soft steady stream of honey flowing from the hive to the queen and back. Honey washes away all cares.

After a while, you may hear a quiet humming sound as you exhale. The bees are happily working in their hive. Inhale to the count of 5 and exhale to the count of 10. Very gradually increase the humming to the count of 20. Deep in the hive, worker bees are digesting honey so that the queen can be nourished and satisfied. The end product is called royal jelly, an energizing food full of predigested B vitamins.

Healing Baths for All Types

One way to calm your voice is with a healing bath that allows the muscles to relax. Soak in a warm bath adding one of these pure essential oils:

- Rosemary or lily of the valley for fatigue or depression
- Hops, vervain, or honeysuckle for anxiety

Vocal and Diction Study

In *The Arts of Beauty,* Lola Montez recommends vocal study for anyone who wishes to arouse the interest of the opposite sex. "The most correct and elegant language loses all its beauty with a bad or ill-trained voice. . . . To be charming in conversation, implies a perfect knowledge of the rare and difficult art of reading."

If your work requires public speaking or presentations, it might be a good idea to get a vocal coach. Proper breathing and vocal production go a long way towards preventing fatigue and nervousness. Lola also recommends reading aloud to "practice the most happy and delightful ideas of soft and appropriate tones." What should you read aloud? Are there good books or plays that you have wanted to see but have not taken the time? If you want to be scientific about it, you might tape your reading and compare yours with the pros.

While learning about phrasing and pacing by reading aloud in a relaxed manner, you might improve your vocal production with a few herbs. A full and easy breath is vital for vocal production.

A Free and Easy Voice

Chinese formulas for digestion and circulation such as Xiao Yao Wan (or Soothing Balance extract, made by Long Hay Flat) have improved breath support for people who have slow digestion or asthma, or for singers who hold tension in the chest and abdomen. A possible substitute is Quiet Digestion made by Health Concerns. You might also make a tea using fresh ginger, mint, tarragon, and lemongrass. A possible homeopathic remedy might be gelsemium 30C, because it eases tension in the solar plexus.

Laryngitis Can Ruin Your Career

One of my clients who sings complains, "Laryngitis has prevented my speaking and singing. It is a disaster." Sometimes laryngitis is the first sign of a cold.

Sometimes it is like a spasm brought on by emotional factors. Homeopathic calc. sulph. 6x can cut short a cold and sore throat because it raises immunity as it cleanses the body. The recommended dose is every 15 minutes during an acute attack.

A Chinese remedy that tastes extremely bitter are tiny pills called Lu Shen Wan. The bottle is the size of a fingernail. It opens clockwise instead of counterclockwise. Everything about it is strange—even the ingredients, which include bovine gallstones. The pills are so bitter tasting that you have to swallow a dose immediately without savoring it. Incredibly, it usually knocks out a dreadful sore throat in less than five minutes.

The quickest and safest way to prevent colds and flu can be found in Chinese herbal medicine. In late 2001, over 100 over-the-counter American-made cold drugs were found to contain a dangerous ingredient, Phenylpropanolamine (commonly called PPA), which has been linked to an estimated 200–500 strokes a year. Some of those medicines for children and adults, which were removed from store shelves, had been on sale for as long as 40 years.

Chinese herbal cold pills work by helping the body to naturally sweat out a cold. They contain natural antibiotic herbs such as honeysuckle flower. Gan Mao Ling, for cold prevention and treatment, and Gan Mao Ching, for flu with fever, are available in Chinese herb shops and supermarkets or online. I list some sources at the back of this book.

A Quick Fix for Vocal Comfort

You can moisturize mouth and throat with a cup or more of American ginseng tea. Its cooling effects increase saliva and prevent chronic thirst. You may want to soak and cook a piece of tremella, known in Chinese supermarkets as white fungus, along with canned corn—like the popular soup sold in Chinese restaurants.

On the other hand, serious or chronic dry lungs, cough, and night sweats can be corrected by taking Tremella and American Ginseng pills from Health Concerns. You might start with 2 tablets to feel the cooling moistening effects. For asthma, bronchitis, chronic viral infections, hot palms and soles and chest, and swollen lymph glands, the dosage can be as high as 3–5 tablets three times daily. Consult with a Chinese herbal expert before using this moistening combination for more than a few days.

You can deepen shallow breath and reverse weakness and chills with a Chinese patent remedy called Ping Chuan Wan, recommended for asthma, emphysema, or shortness of breath. The normal dosage is 6 pills three times daily between meals. Possible substitutes include a pinch of thyme and clove added to a cup of tea.

Practice one of the breathing exercises from this chapter for 15 minutes twice during the day. Or lie flat and relaxed on your back, stretch in both directions with feet and head, then relax. Repeat this several times until the back feels longer. Place both hands on the navel and inhale gently into the lower abdomen. Make sure to relax muscles from the head to the feet with each breath. Exhale gently through your feet. Very quietly hiss a sound as you exhale, but do not engage your voice. Relax your throat and imagine that the sound is coming from your abdomen. Gradually try to extend the length of your exhalation.

Especially for Men

A low-pitched voice is cultivated by many men as well as women. In TCM, vocal pitch and timbre is a sign of the heart's health and circulation. Vocal strain is aggravated by pollution and smoking. Antistress herbs such as gotu kola and kava gradually sooth nervousness, but many people require special help for smoking and pollution.

Lo han kuo, a Chinese herb recommended for dry lungs or dry cough, can be used as a tea or coffee sweetener. Lo han kuo, which resembles a round, dry, hollow brown pod, comes as an ingredient in several Chinese chong ji (instant beverages) recommended for cough and skin blemishes. One of my favorites, available online, is called Beverage of Lo Han Kuo Zhenzhu & Sheshecao. It contains—aside from lo han kuo—skullcap, asparagus, *Oldenlandia diffus* (bai hua sheshecao), and powdered pearls. The combination is an antipyretic salivant, thirst quencher that is also recommended for reducing rheumatism, carbuncles, and the ill-effects of pollution. The label reads, "this beverage sleeks the sexual organs." I think they mean it's diuretic. Women can use it too.

Lola's Way

The natural voice is an expression of the body's ease and the heart's pleasure. In order to have full breath capacity, you need to be relaxed yet actively involved. Deepening your breath will increase oxygen intake, reduce fatigue, and help prevent cloudy thinking.

You need to have strong legs to breathe well. Your vocal support does not originate in the throat but in the legs. To strengthen balance, try walking backward as boxers do during training. It engages muscles that you have probably never used. Inhale and exhale slowly as you visually fix a distant point at the horizon. Of course, I don't recommend doing this in subway stations. I enjoy walking backward on a deserted country road. Pick a quiet time and a place that has no pollution.

Morning Wake-up Visualization

Stand tall but relaxed. Imagine that your head is a large yellow sunflower basking in the sunshine. Your roots stretch deep into the earth. Inhale through the flower and exhale down through the thick roots.

With your fingertips, gently massage small circles along the hairline, on the temples, around eyes and ears, along the jaw bone, and around the mouth. Very lightly tap your fingertips as though drumming on a tabletop on your forehead, cheek bones, and around the mouth. This encourages lymph drainage. Either with a skin brush or the palms of both hands, gently massage yourself from head to foot: massage along the sides of the neck, over tops of shoulders, and down the arms. Press at the underarms and massage around breasts, down the sides of the ribs, and down the abdomen to the groin. Massage the thighs and include the front and back of the knees. Press the sides of the calves down to the ankles. Massage ankles and feet, including the toes.

Stand and stretch your spine and arms up toward the ceiling, spreading the fingers like leaves. Then touch the palms together in front of your chest. Relax your back and let the shoulders drop. Plant your feet into the earth and breathe down to your roots for 10 breaths.

Evening Relaxing Beauty Visualization

In a tub of warm water or lying flat in bed, imagine every part of your face in the following manner: as you inhale gently into the lower abdomen, picture the part of your face to wish to relax. As you exhale, mentally tell that part to relax and let it melt to the earth.

Imagine that your face is a water lily floating on a tranquil pond. The lovely petals are smooth and soft. Its fragrance is delicious. Your hair melts into the water. A white swan floats from your forehead to touch your lungs, abdomen, and legs down to your toes. Your eyes rest like pearls inside the soft cushions of a shell. They sink through your body into the water. Your ears are shiny green leaves in the water. Your cheeks and mouth are a floating tropical garden of ripe fruit and flowers that falls to your chest, lower abdomen, legs, and feet. Your face is a lotus flower whose green and brown stems touch the bottom of the pond. Your feet wriggle in warm mud as fish play around you.

Attitude Training

Even if you never sing or act professionally, you will want your voice to convey the confidence and ease of a professional. Voice training arms us with breath control, stamina, and focus. Another essential thing for any voice is to step aside and let the God in the music touch the listener. No matter what the repertoire, the voice communicates heart to heart. Maria Callas, during her master classes at Julliard, spoke of being "generous" with the voice. More than vocal culture, she taught me what a great lady does. On stage and off, be guided by your character and your voice. Your every emotion should sound beautiful. When angry, soften your face, take a breath, plant your feet, throw back your head, and laugh like a diva. Confidence and skill work better than losing your temper.

An Assignment:

I dare you: ask someone who has never seen you to describe your appearance after listening to your voice. No matter if you are a phone salesperson or a radio personality, have your listeners describe you in detail—your height, weight, hair color, clothing—everything particular about your style. You may learn something surprising about your image from their description.

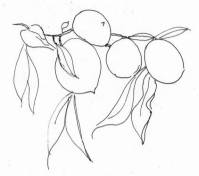

PART FOUR

Beauty Karma

"Come, my friends,
'Tis not too late to seek a newer world . . .
To sail beyond the sunset and the baths
Of all the western stars"
            —*Ulysses*, Alfred Lord Tennyson

17

Beauty Survival Skills

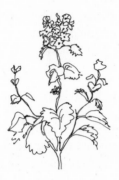

"An attack on New York, the city of the 21st Century, is an
attack on our values, on who we are as a people."
—SENATOR HILLARY RODHAM CLINTON

With these words, United States senator from New York, Hillary Clinton—
America's most famous woman, and quite possibly a future president—has
succinctly expressed our unity as a people. The assault on September 11, 2001
was aimed at something fundamentally cultural and aesthetic. New York
accepts all traditions and all aspects of beauty from porn to haute couture.
New York represents the multicultural, multiracial promise of a greater America. However, to be alive in a time of war is stressful and harms beauty.

This chapter covers remedies for anxiety, injury, toxic pollution, and
related beauty issues. It is especially helpful for people living in and working
under hazardous conditions such as those in construction, military and police
personnel, medical professionals, and the clergy. A definite plus for all is
that detoxifying treatments naturally improve energy, breathing, complexion,
and mood.

Adrift on a Sea of Troubles

Faced with an emotional shock or serious illness, many people turn to drinking, smoking, or drug use. Weakened, they victimize themselves. Depressed people typically neglect their looks. Protecting health and natural beauty gives you an advantage: in the process of looking better, you help yourself to overcome emotional trauma. Creating healthy beauty is an antiterrorist act.

The Chinese have a long history as survivors. Wars, plagues, and natural catastrophes over the centuries have spurred them to create their elaborate medicine. If you have suffered a harsh blow, such as the loss of a loved one, you may feel adrift on a sea of uncertainty, questioning all you do and stand for. You need to see and seize your future.

Your Vision for the Future

For visionary dreams, Chinese Taoist sages drank warm yuan zhi (*Polygala tenuifolia*) tea before bed. Polygala root is said to calm the spirit and ease the flow of qi (energy circulation) to the heart. Useful for insomnia, palpitations with anxiety, restlessness, and mental confusion, it releases pent-up feelings as it clears mucus congestion in the lungs. Steep ½ teaspoon of the powdered herb per cup of boiling water.

Begin now in developing skills for achieving inner peace. Your training will surface when you need it. Tai chi and qi gong movements are designed to enhance life force. Practiced regularly, they develop smooth muscle action, balance, agility, grace, strength, deep breathing, and mental focus. Chinese movement practices such as these, often done to stay trim, are powerful crisis-intervention methods. Practice them during extreme stress. Deliberate breathing and slow movements moderate fight-or-flight patterns that muddle your chances of survival. Here is a daily exercise useful for preventing and treating panic.

A Relaxation Exercise

Sit with your back against a chair and keep both feet flat, or lie on your back in bed. Breathe gently into the lower abdomen. Your chest should not move up and down. Put your hands on your lower abdomen at the navel. As you inhale, fill yourself with light and warmth. Imagine a flame. With each exhalation, melt tension from head to foot. Don't skip over anything. The heart, liver, stomach, and intestines all need to relax. When emotions arise, melt them too. You will feel muscle spasms release as blood flows smoothly through your body. Your hands and feet may feel warmer.

To warm and relax your entire body, use sesame oil for a foot massage or soak your feet in sage tea. To cool the body and reduce fever, soak feet with warm water and organic lemon juice. Detoxify from environmental pollution and bad habits with a daily 20-minute bath adding 2 cups to 1 quart of apple cider vinegar to hot water.

Mental Focus Quick

When you are upset, does your heart race? Does your mind go blank? Signs of anxiety improve quickly with homeopathic remedies. I have already discussed homeopathic gelsemium 30C and aconite 30C used for anxiety and panic. Combining them calms an emotional tidal wave of fear. During times of prolonged stress, add 10 pills of each to 1 quart of spring water and sip it throughout the day between meals. Take a thermos with you when you fly.

Shock and Emotional Stress

Do you feel faint from stress or after an emotional shock? To revive yourself or another person from sleepiness or feeling faint, press the acupuncture point located at the bottom of the nose between the nostrils. Pushing gently upward towards the hairline with the length of your finger or the length of a pencil sends blood to the brain, which awakens the senses. It is one of the areas acupuncturists use to revive a person from a coma. Other points used to normalize circulation are located about 1 inch above the inside of the wrist between the tendons. Massage the hands and feet until they are warm and show improved blood circulation.

A safe and effective natural form of smelling salts is real, edible camphor, found in Chinese or East Indian herb shops. Use only the healthy, nonsynthetic camphor, which is often used in Chinese heart remedies to dilate blood vessels. Store some in an empty cosmetic jar in your car to keep yourself awake while driving. A small pinch placed in each nostril awakens the senses. Avoid swallowing it. Keep a person in shock quiet and warm. Speak gently and calmly. A few drops by mouth of homeopathic Rescue Remedy is recommended to help bring about physical balance after an accident or shock.

A Detoxifying Beauty Treatment that Awakens Senses

One pinch of natural edible camphor or one drop of Australian Tea Tree Oil, applied with a Q-tip to the inside of the nose, clears sinus congestion, eye irritations, or mental fuzziness resulting from pollution, chemicals, and dust. They make eyes water. If the treatment burns from sores inside the nose, use a dab of aloe vera gel at the same time. If you spend time in an environment where you suspect anthrax, asbestos, or chemical weapons, keep a little aloe vera gel in your nose to prevent deep inhalation. Ayurvedic doctors recommend aloe gel in the nose as a beauty treatment for red or swollen eyes, thinning head hair, and bad temper! Its cooling, detoxifying effects are quickly absorbed by the brain when placed in the nose.

Injury

Yunnan Paiyao (powder and capsules), a first-aid herbal remedy carried by every Chinese soldier, combines pungent antiseptic herbs such as myrrh and tienchi ginseng. It stops hemorrhage and is recommended for gunshot wounds, puncture wounds, and surgery. It heals damaged blood vessels and normalizes bleeding.

Yunnan Paiyao is known for reducing pain, bruising, and swelling as well as bleeding. Noted New York plastic surgeon Dr. Gerald Ginsberg has enthusiastically praised Yunnan Paiyao for its ability to reduce bleeding during surgery and liposuction. Take the small red pill before surgery then follow up with 4–6 capsules daily until circulation and wounds are healed and bruising, pain, and swelling are reduced.

Chronic Oozing Wounds

Yunnan Paiyao resolves slow-healing or oozing wounds fast by bringing pus to the surface and drying and disinfecting wetness. It works well for insect and animal bites. Pour on the powder locally and take capsules according to the recommended dosage. For information on Yunnan Paiyao for internal problems, including menstrual flooding, chronic gastritis, and bleeding ulcers, see *Asian Health Secrets*.

Chest Discomforts

Smoke inhalation and physical or emotional stress can make your chest ache and your heart weak. A number of Chinese herbs work fast to reestablish heart rhythm and circulation. Chinese Revival Pills come in a tiny porcelain vase easily kept in your pocket. They combine edible camphor and ligustrum, which respectively dilate blood vessels and stimulate chest circulation. Depending on the dosage, the tiny pills are used for chronic or acute chest pain. You can sniff them as smelling salts or take 4 pills twice daily to prevent heart discomfort. Have your Chinese herbalist show them to you. The pills are a wise office remedy. Also see Yin/Yang Sisters Breathe Free instant beverage, discussed in this chapter.

Instant Beverages for Home and Office

To increase resistance and vitality, Yin/Yang Sisters brand has developed eight concentrated powdered herbal beverages. I have recommended these high-quality herbal products in chapters concerning seasonal allergies and energy problems, the voice, complexion, and rejuvenation. They can be served hot or cold and sweetened with a Chinese sugar substitute such as Sheshecao crystals.

To clear the body of impurities and enhance natural resistance to dangerous pollution, keep the following Yin/Yang Sister Brand Instant Beverages on hand: Gorgeous You, Clean Habits, Breathe Free, and Happy Garden Tea. Don't be misled by their whimsical names. The manufacturer in Jiangsu, China, normally supplies hospitals with herbal medicines. The ingredients are all top-quality organic herbs packaged for the Western consumer. Each dose is individually foil-wrapped to protect freshness and potency. They all improve appearance.

Gorgeous You contains tonic herbs recommended to build vitality for weakened conditions ranging from simple exhaustion to AIDS. The ingredients enhance blood production, energy, and circulation, which are beneficial for skin and hair. Clean Habits is a powerful liver and blood cleanser that reduces blemishes. Breathe Free improves sinus congestion and is useful for reducing the negative effects of airborne germs and pollution. Happy Garden Tea is recommended for depression, anxiety, and certain menopausal symptoms.

Lin Sisters Herb Shop, in New York's Chinatown, recommends Breathe Free and Gorgeous You as daily beverages for asthma and sinus congestion. They have become especially popular since September 11. They are best taken with hot water between meals, and one dose daily is considered appropriate for prevention. Higher doses are sometimes required for treatment.

Blood-Cleansing Herbs and Itchy Rashes

Complexion-marring diseases require potent liver- and blood-cleansing, antiinflammatory herbs. Such herbs are described by Chinese doctors as having the ability to "clear fire poisons." Acidic foods, alcohol, cigarettes, chemical pollution, and epidemic germs lead to fevers, skin inflammation, and infection ("fire poisons"). Complexion issues that can be improved with blood-cleansing herbs include carbuncles and nasty red and itchy sores. Blood-cleansing herbs do not allow germs, impurities, and inflammation to remain in the body. An herbal antigerm regime may mark the beginning of your campaign to stop smoking and drinking. The eventual result can be a milky-smooth complexion.

An inexpensive Chinese herbal antibiotic is Chuan Xin Lian pills, which contain concentrated andrographis, dandelion, and isatis—two antibiotic herbs and a blood cleanser. It is recommended for swollen glands, blemishes, fevers, infections, sore throat and gums, and mumps. The normal dosage is 2 pills three times daily with water. The dosage can be increased as needed without side effects. Reduce dosage if diarrhea occurs. You might combine 3 Chuan Xin Lian pills along with 4 pills of Lien Chiao Pai Tu Pien twice daily between meals to cool and cleanse blemishes. You can easily combine these pills with Yin/Yang Sisters Clean Habits, a liver- and blood-cleanser beverage. If cleansing weakens vitality, add Gorgeous You instant beverage as needed. Taking these precautions, you will have a better chance to resist fire poisons and have radiant skin.

I have never heard a traditional Chinese herbalist recommend acidophilus (or yogurt) for improving digestion after using antibiotic herbs. Normally, they recommend tonic herbs such as astragalus (one of the ingredients in Gorgeous You). However, if your digestion suffers from herbal cleansers, especially if cramps and bloating occur, I recommend 1–2 capsules of acidophilus daily.

Beauty Treatments in a Pinch

My friend, Michelle, who is an officer in the Army National Guard, spent time in Kohbar, Kuwait, during the Persian Gulf War. She suffered skin outbreaks from chemicals that lined her protective clothing. She had no cosmetics with her but found a few foods that were helpful when applied as a mask. Facial treatments made with acidic foods cleanse, exfoliate, and heal skin. The following washes and masks may not be luxurious, but they work well under extreme conditions.

- Cleanse face, body, and teeth with brewed tea. Tannic acid from tea steeped longer than 20 minutes reduces burns and skin irritations. Tea is antiseptic and speeds healing.
- Mash a very ripe papaya (exfoliant) and apply it as a mask for 20 minutes. If you can't find fresh ingredients, crush papaya pills and add water.
- Mix 1 tablespoon of honey, 1 teaspoon of canned cranberry sauce, and ½ teaspoon of cornmeal for a deep-cleansing facial scrub. Acids in the honey and cranberries remove dead skin, shrink pores, and brighten complexion. Cornmeal exfoliates. Leave it on for 3–5 minutes, massage lightly with wet fingers, and remove it with warm water. For sensitive skin, omit the cornmeal.
- Nourish dry skin with finely chopped fresh or dried greens, such as watercress, alfalfa sprouts, dandelion, or parsley. Steep them in very hot water and apply the pulp to your face for 10–15 minutes. For extra dry skin, add a few drops of corn, sunflower, or olive oil. Remove the green

mask with water, and rub face and neck with sliced raw peeled potato, an exfoliant high in potassium.

- An antibiotic mask that improves acne blemishes and herpes discomforts can be made by adding a little hot water to Yin/Yang Sisters Clean Habits. It contains skullcap, isatis, red peony root, gentian root, gardenia fruit, and licorice root.

My suggestion if you live in any highly polluted area is to grow sprouts (see page 42). You feel as though you are gardening when growing organic sunflower seeds, lentils, or fenugreek sprouts in a plastic bag stuck into your knapsack or in a jar laid on its side in your desk drawer. Drain and rinse them daily with fresh water. In a couple of days, you will have sprouts rich in vitamin E and nutrients for skin and hair health and beauty.

On the Beat

Laurie is a petite, pretty New York cop, who is rarely recognized as one. Once, late at night, an uptight deli cashier accused her of stealing something. She was dressed in tight jeans, a skimpy halter top, and big afro haircut. She smiled, shook her head, and opened her sling purse to show her badge and gun.

Laurie spends long hours on her beat in cars or walking. Fast foods, sometimes the only thing she can find, give her indigestion. Homeopathic carbo veg. 30C, made from charcoal, absorbs gas and eases digestion. To be most effective, observe a few food combining rules: never mix fruit with protein or starch. Fruit slows digestion and causes gas. If you can only eat one thing, make it a vegetable instead of fruit. Wait at least 20 minutes after eating then take a dose of homeopathic carbo veg. 30C. If you need a second dose, take it after another 15 minutes and continue until you get relief.

Coffee causes cramps and irritability. Aspirin, recommended far too often for pain and as a blood thinner, can cause serious gastrointestinal tract irritation and bleeding. Flat (noncarbonated) water and tea do not upset digestion or cause indigestion bubbles.

A Quick Fix Beauty Survival Kit

A few simple remedies for fatigue, infections, toxins, and emotional upset are wise to keep on hand at home and at work. They include homeopathic remedies and herbal instant beverages. You can use them at the same time as long as they are recommended for the same sort of discomfort. For example, gelsemium 30C with Happy Garden Tea, or pulsatilla 30C with Breathe Free. There is one exception: do not combine homeopathic aconite 30C with any other remedy, food, coffee, or toothpaste.

Homeopathic Remedies

Gelsemium 30C: for lethargy, self doubt, anxiety, and weakness

Pulsatilla 30C: for weeping, sadness, and thick, bland mucus congestion

Aconite 30C: for fear, hysteria, and high fever with headache

Belladonna 30C: for hot throbbing pains and burning ear and throat infections

Mercury 30C: for infections with pus, perspiration, saliva or discharges that smell bad, accompanied by fever (for use longer than three days, consult a professional)

Yin/Yang Sisters Instant Beverages

Happy Garden Tea: for worry, depression, insomnia, and menopausal stress

Breathe Free: for sinus congestion and breathing

Clean Habits: for liver cleansing, blemishes, pollution, fevers, headaches, and rash

Gorgeous You: for aging, sallow skin, poor circulation, and low enthusiasm and energy

Flu Away: for cold and flu symptoms, rhinitis, aches, sore throat, and fever

Especially for Men

A lot of men hold tension in the shoulders, abdomen, and groin. They may want to strike at an enemy but refrain. They may sit all day to make them stiff. Neck vertebrae may be out of place from whiplash or arms painful or numb from carpal tunnel syndrome. The result is that their shoulders feel like lead bars.

Abdominal bloating and indigestion are made worse by stress. Groin pain can result from hip or nerve problems, pent-up frustration, and poor circulation. The groin is on the pathway for the liver acupuncture meridian, a channel involved with sexual vitality and aggression. Acting out aggression is not always advised, but using herbs to free circulation is.

Health Concerns makes Ease 2 pills for reducing neck and shoulder pain, muscle tension, and gastrointestinal disorders, including loose bowels. The formula contains bupleurum, pueraria, pinellia, cinnamon, peony, ginseng, scute, licorice, and ginger. Ordering Health Concerns remedies requires a visit or an e-mail to an herbalist. You can e-mail me at lethah@earthlink.net.

Lola's Way

Why use sugar when there is something better! Ban Lan Gen Chongji is an instant beverage made from Baphicacanthus cusia or Isatis tinctoria (a.k.a. isatis, wild indigo). An herbal antibiotic, it cools and clears skin irritations and reduces fevers and sore throats. This Chinese instant beverage made from 70% indigo root, 25% indigo leaf, and 5% cane sugar is sweet enough to use as a sugar substitute. The original dried herb, banlangen, is very bitter. It is a powerful remedy used in China for fever, infections, hepatitis, malaria, and meningitis because it is highly detoxifying for the entire body, especially the blood.

However, Ban Lan Gen Chongji is milder in action and pleasant tasting to use on a daily basis. Add one serving to a pot of tea or in cooking. The remedy helps to clear rashes as it protects the liver against possible irritants such as pollution, germs, and chemical poisons. This beverage is recommended for children of all ages who love sweets.

Hopefully, you will never need these remedies to prevent and cure the effects of toxic pollution or warfare. You can use any of them, however, as safe, effective cleansers. A practical daily cleansing routine including instant beverages such as Clean Habits and Breathe Free is the first step toward rejuvenation.

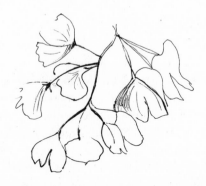

18

Look Young, Feel Young

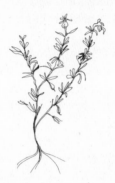

> "She behaves as if she was beautiful. Most American
> women do. It is the secret of their charm."
> —OSCAR WILDE

During the summer of 2001, Bill Maher, the host of ABC's "Politically Incorrect," greeted his television guest Michael York with, "You look better than ever." He might have said *younger* than ever. Born in Fulmer, England, the handsome actor began his movie career in the 1960s when director Franco Zeffirelli chose him to play Tybalt in *Romeo and Juliet.* His impetuous D'Artagnan in *The Three Musketeers* (1974) set the scene for romantic leads featuring his youthful appeal. His popularity has remained fresh and growing. A new crop of fans love him in pop favorites such as *Austin Powers: The Spy Who Shagged Me* (1999). Michael has delighted audiences in over 112 movies and has written *Accidentally on Purpose*, *A Shakespearean Actor Prepares,* and *Dispatches from Armageddon.*

I think a major factor in his appeal is his spiritual awareness. It would be difficult to find someone more respectful of others. Michael is still a true Oxford gentleman. He treats everyone with consideration. His genuineness and integrity show through in all his characters.

Michael's warm, resonant voice, a trademark, is one result of his text-based approach to acting. In *A Shakespearean Actor Prepares*, he recommends studying a role this way: "If you read the speech aloud, paying attention to the suggested breaks, the key words and heavy stresses, you will probably find a patrician fury welling up inside you—almost of its own accord." Careful preparation allows the actor to remain sensitive and open to experimentation. Openness and a creative attitude keep us young.

I asked Jacquie Jordan, a Los Angeles-based daytime television producer, what she considered most attractive in actors. She smiled: "Professionals who are natural, bountiful, and lovely to work with. The camera doesn't lie. You need to be yourself. Celebrities who are relaxed in their own skin are beautiful. They are always finding new ways to keep themselves challenged and excited."

This chapter provides "extreme beauty" rejuvenation techniques that work faster than ordinary methods. I hope they keep you challenged and excited.

Stop Smoking Now!

Many jobs can be hazardous to your health. One of my internet clients works at the bottom of a mine, where temperatures soar over 120 degrees. He says, "Miners can cook eggs without a stove, and sometimes their clothes melt." Other people work in beauty salons, where hair dyes and sprays make their eyes wince, and they may develop a cough and chronic thirst. Truck and cab drivers can't escape dangerous fumes. Their jobs damage their lung health, and because of this their vitality is drained. These people suffer because they need their jobs to survive. They cannot give up their jobs as easily as you can stop smoking.

Lung irritation underlies anxiety. Stress, pollution, and prescription medicines rampage inside us as the sun increases their effects. We need to cleanse, cool, and nourish our lungs to prevent aging. When you quit smoking, your lungs can be rejuvenated and your complexion can be clear and moist. Smoking stains your fingers, fouls your breath, and costs money. Do you need more reasons to quit?

Helpful Lung-Moistening Foods

All sorts of green vegetables—kale, parsley, watercress, endive, dandelion, chicory or cooked spinach, okra, asparagus—as well as berries, cherries, peaches, apples, and cooked oatmeal help to cleanse and prepare your body for positive change.

Don't try to quit a long-standing habit all at once. Your body is addicted to smoking even if your mind is not. Smoking involves your hands, your face, and your body language. It becomes part of your style. You might try chewing cinnamon or licorice sticks when your hands reach for a cigarette. The lungs and heart both suffer from smoking; cinnamon helps circulation and licorice is moistening and refreshing. You also need to free trapped emotions. Chest tightness, from cholesterol and emotional stress, is eased with improved circulation.

A Chinese Pill for Improved Circulation

One useful Chinese patent remedy for chest discomfort is Dan Shen Wan. The pills combine salvia (red Chinese sage) to energize the heart and prepared camphor to help dilate blood vessels. A dose of 4 pills three times daily is recommended to prevent or treat angina (chest pain). You may need to take extra cordyceps extract, which dilates the aorta in times of stress.

Clean Habits for Preventing Withdrawal Symptoms

Homeopathic nux vomica 30C taken between meals either five times daily or as needed (every 15 minutes) can ease and prevent cravings for addictions as well as stress discomforts, including headache, nausea, palpitations, and sinus congestion.

Clean Habits Instant Beverage is safe and effective after celebrations (or anytime) to deep cleanse the liver and blood from addictive eating, drinking, and smoking. It combines cleansing and calming herbs along with digestive herbs so that withdrawal symptoms such as headache, irritability, and nervousness are reduced. You can enjoy it daily by adding one or two packages to an 8-ounce glass of apple juice. It refreshes both body and mind. The ingredients are completely caffeine-free (gentian, skullcap, gardenia buds, isatis root, red poria, and licorice root).

Gentian is a bitter liver cleanser that supports breathing and is recommended to reduce depression. Dr. Yves Requena, author and TCM doctor practicing in Aix en Provence, France, recommends gentian to "strengthen the spleen," which ensures better vitamin absorption and less spaciness and water retention. Skullcap reduces nervousness and eye aches. Gardenia buds reduce mucus congestion and infectious discharges from eyes, nose, throat and elsewhere in the body. Isatis (wild indigo; in Chinese ban lan gan) is an antimicrobial that quells fevers from malaria. It is used for encephalitis in China. Poria is diuretic. Red poria refers to the outer shell of the dried herb also has nervine qualities. The herb is cleansing and balancing for the urinary tract and nervous system. Licorice is added to reduce digestive discomforts.

Better Breathing and Clean Breath

Licorice root tea has its fans among herbalists, but it comes with warnings. Licorice is a demulcent, which means it moistens and allows thick mucus congestion to soften. However, if you have thick ankles, retain water anywhere in the body, or have hypertension, do not drink licorice tea alone. It is safer in herbal combinations. Otherwise, it might increase water retention. I think licorice works better for chest and abdominal discomfort if you add a slice of dried citrus peel (chen pi) and three cloves to a cup of licorice tea. The stimulating spices help resolve mucus.

Detoxification programs sometimes unleash chronic problems. Sinus allergies and post-nasal drip can make life miserable. Breathe Free, the Yin/Yang Sisters beverage, helps clear your senses so you can enjoy life. Breathe Free can be combined with an antimucus diet low in dairy foods and sweets. Drinking Clean Habits after meals and Breathe Free between meals will help you to eliminate a hacking, rumbling smoker's cough and bad breath.

Dr. Tieraona Low Dog, a stunning American Indian herbalist, midwife, biochemist, and family physician, is medical director of the Treehouse Center of Integrative Medicine in Albuquerque, New Mexico, as well as a member of the faculty for Columbia University's Botanical Medicine in Modern Clinical Practice annual May conference. Her long, flowing raven hair and warm, look-you-straight-eagle-in-the-eye manner remind me of Western paintings of desert maidens on prancing horses. Dr. Low Dog, who describes herself as a "doctor AND a mom," becomes personally involved with entire families in her private practice. Her patients know and love herbs.

Stress-Related Cramps and Cold Sores

Tieraona's herbal remedies are no-frills, fast-acting, and very effective. For cramps from indigestion and stress, she often recommends a brew of catnip, fennel, and chamomile tea. For cold sores or herpes fever blisters, she recommends topical application of lemon balm extract as well as drinking licorice tea.

You can cool irritations by adding cleansing and moistening herbs to your daily routine. Your skin will show the difference soon. If you want to make fast progress, acupuncture usually works to stop smoking within three to seven treatments. Then you can calculate the sum of money you will save by not smoking. Put the savings aside as a travel fund, and you may get to Hawaii before you know it!

Rejuvenate with Breath and Movement

Linda van Horn teaches applied chair and floor Hatha yoga to reverse aging and enhance healthy beauty. Retired from the beauty profession after running her own salon in New York, she decided to heal herself in the best ways possible with a vegetarian diet, Japanese massage, and meditative qi gong and yoga movements. "For years I stood like this," she said jutting one hip out and balancing her weight on one leg as she mimed blow-drying some-one's hair. Poor posture and whiplash damaged her neck, spine, and hip with chronic nerve pain and arthritis. After years of re-educating her body, she is one of the most beautiful and graceful women I know. Breath, movements, diet, meditation, and a few herbs (such as myrrh capsules as needed for arthritis discomfort and gotu kola tea for nerve health) keep Linda young and pain free.

Linda's great gift to her many loyal fans, aside from her calming presence and sugar-cane Jamaican accent, is a simple daily stretch routine designed to rejuvenate the back, legs, and face. It also reduces wrinkles.

The Child Pose

Get out of your chair. Go on to your knees then fold your legs under you and sit on your shins. Breathe into the lower abdomen. As you exhale, bend forward toward the opposite wall lowering your body and head as close to the floor as easily possible. This releases air and tension from the abdominal area and opens the pelvis and spine for deeper breath. When you can manage it, make two fists. Put one on top of the other onto the floor in front of you. Lower your head to rest on your fists. You will look completely doubled over, collapsed on your shins. Stay there breathing comfortably like a baby in the womb in order to release tension along the spine. Stay there as long as you like. To get up, gently reverse the movements. Inhale as you sit up.

Chair Yoga

If you work sitting, try to keep your knees higher than the groin to relax the back and discourage water retention pain in the legs. Seated in your chair, lift, bounce, or move your legs as though walking until any tension disappears.

Make a wide 70-degree angle with your legs open and feet firmly placed on the floor. Inhale, then lift your spine, neck, head, and arms up out of the chair towards the ceiling. As you exhale, reach forward towards the opposite wall and bend over to hang in front of you. Clasp your elbows with the opposite hands. The blood will rush to your face. Your pelvis and spine will feel open. Breathe normally and relaxed.

Breast Beauty and Health

According to the American Cancer Society, China holds the world's best record for breast health. Their traditional medicine promotes the use of neither mammograms nor synthetic hormones. However, Chinese women have numerous methods for promoting breast beauty and health at home and in Chinese beauty shops. Special herbal teas increase circulation to enhance breast firmness. Herbal patches worn against the body or sewn into under-garments, breast massage, acupuncture, magnets, and energy work are used to reduce mastitis (painful swollen breasts) and fibroids. In China, women go to inexpensive public clinics to receive treatments especially suited to their condition in order to dissolve lumps and cysts. In Chinese beauty shops here and abroad, you can find breast stimulater machines and herbal creams to enhance bust size.

The following recommendations apply for men and women who want to improve circulation, muscle tone, and reduce the threat of fibroids. Remember: Men get breast cancer too. Some women opt for breast surgery to alter their bust size, which can lead to complications. The following methods to ease circulation are *always* healing and beautifying.

An Exercise to Lift the Breast

Strengthening chest muscles can help lift the bust and improve circulation. Susie, a former publishing executive, trims her hedges with old-fashioned clippers instead of electric shears. She demonstrated placing her arms in a circle as if holding a beach ball then thrusted them inward against resistance. "Sometimes I pull a thick exercise rubber band to make the resistance. You place the long rubber band across your back, hold each end in your hands and pull them towards each other in the front." She beams: "After overcoming breast cancer, I believe in everything natural—foods, herbs, fresh water and air, and exercise."

A Homeopathic Breast Beauty Cream

To enhance circulation, ease post-surgery discomforts, and help prevent fibroids, I recommend homeopathic arnica ointment or cream as a breast massage treatment. The homeopathic remedy is recommended for bruises, painful muscles, and swelling from injuries. However, it helps poor circulation anywhere. Arnica ointments and creams found in health-food stores are usually greaseless and will not stain clothing. Apply the cream to the entire breast after a bath or shower and wear it under clothing to enhance circulation and reduce discomfort. One Chinese doctor I heard about used direct electrostimulation to reduce fibroids. His patient, an angry American woman, stopped after one treatment because her bra size increased. I prefer the homeopathic cream to enhance breast circulation. It is safer and you can do it at home.

Daily Herbs for Breast Well-Being

When I studied acupuncture and Chinese herbal remedies for breast cancer some years ago in a Shanghai hospital, a doctor with 40 years of experience told me, "Breast health is damaged by low metabolism, faulty circulation, hormone imbalances, as well as anxiety, grief, and melancholy that retard general vitality. Synthetic drug medicines create what TCM doctors call 'stagnant qi' poor energy circulation.That also impairs vitality and circulation."

Certain herbs can help eliminate underlying toxins as they improve circulation throughout the body. For example, daily capsules of dandelion and myrrh are very beneficial for circulation on a long-term basis. Take at least twice as many dandelion capsules as myrrh, for example, 6 dandelion and 3 myrrh twice daily. They also cleanse the uterus.

Breast beauty means more than the absence of fibroids. It engages our feelings of sexual allure and feeling at ease with our body. Troubled emotions especially interfere with circulation in the chest and breast tissue because they are close to the heart. Improving circulation and mood with Happy Garden Tea can help take the load off your chest.

Nature's Vortex

I never used a magnet to pick up nails as a kid in school. Instead, I discovered magnets after developing chronic back and wrist pain from writing books. Magnets pull information off credit cards and writing off computer discs. They also pull muscle tension out of your body with an energy vortex that swirls away pain. Rite Aid and CVS pharmacies sell magnets made into waist bands, wrist straps, knee guards, and shoulder coverings. You can feel positively magnetic! Small individual spot magnets are placed as needed on fingers or stressed muscles. Manufacturers warn against using magnets if you have a pacemaker or serious heart irregularities. We will use magnets, and their herbal equivalent, to reshape the body with renewed circulation.

Dr. M. G. Zhu of Shanghai Magnet & Biotech Co., Ltd, located at No. 16 Qunyu Road in the Jiading district in Shanghai, China, offered in an e-mail to send me a couple of hundred "MAGIC painless acupuncture magnetic plasters" for my patients. The magnetic plasters are actually aromatic herbal patches used for the treatment of aches, mammary disease, hypertension, and asthma. The dime-sized patches are pasted on to acupuncture points or painful areas for painless acupuncture therapy (see www.magic-magnet.com).

On my shoulder, the dime-sized patches felt hot—not from the patch, but from the force of my energy moving through a numb arm. The next day, my arm felt better. Eureka! Why not use magnets and herbal patches for facelifts, breast beauty, and cellulite treatments? Enhanced circulation tightens sluggish muscle tone and sagging skin.

Be careful when treating tender breast tissue. Tapes used to cover magnets and herbal patches can hurt when removed. I would use a nonsticky magnet or the lymph drainage treatment I describe later. Place magnets for several hours or overnight around breast lumps or the dark skin around the nipple. Never place magnets over the heart, and limit the use of magnets to several days a week. Magnet mavens inform me that circulation becomes accustomed to magnets. Their effects are diminished if used daily. The same goes for magnet pads under bed sheets and magnets used in shoes.

Magnets and Herbal Patches for Leg Muscle Tone

Regular slimming and toning treatments with electrostimulation or lasers can maintain muscle tone for a longer, sleeker you. If you can afford it, a weekly trip to New York's Greenwich Village to see Tracie Martyn and her slimming machine ($150 per hour) gives quick, temporary results. You may bump into Uma Thurman, Naomi Campbell, or Meg Ryan, who also visit. In Beverly Hills, Thibiant Spa has a Seaweed Anti-Cellulite Detox Envelopment ($125) using spirulina and fucus seaweeds. You might get a slightly less expensive Fat Zap Wrap ($100) at one of the Sports Club/LA in Los Angeles or New York.

I have developed a stimulation technique for home use. Most stimulation treatments aim for deep muscle insertion points at big joints in order to lengthen and tone muscles. For example, the muscle insertion points for the thighs are found at the knees and hip joints. To help flatten the abdomen, the best points are located above the groin, under the ribs, and near the top of the knees. For the buttocks, we stimulate the waist, the tailbone, and the creases under the buttocks, behind the knees, and at the middle of the calf.

Seaweed wraps and slimming creams work only skin deep. Their effects vary. Magnets, which emit a subtle current, act deeply and last longer. You can stimulate select acupuncture points using a variety of means. This enhances the body's natural energy currents to improve circulation and eliminate fatigue and water retention that maintain fat and cellulite bumps.

How to Use Magnets at Home

When I see private clients, I observe their general health and energy level by taking their pulse and examining their tongue like a Chinese herbalist. Here are some general rules to follow when using anti-fat stimulation or muscle-toning methods:

- Avoid electrostimulation and magnets if you have heart problems or severe depression. If you have high blood pressure, consult an expert.
- Avoid electrostimulation if you are sick or pregnant. Good times for treatments include before and after events that might retard circulation, such as surgery, traveling, and menstrual periods. Stimulate more frequently if your work involves hours of sitting or standing.
- Place magnets at large joints for 30 minutes twice daily

Wearing a TheraP magnetic waistband next to the skin increases local perspiration. That helps with slimming. Place magnets or herbal patches (or have electrostimulation) on areas that encourage muscle tone, like around large joints such as hips and knees. When you place the magnets it will look as though you are making a ring around each leg at the hip. Do the same for each knee using magnets above the kneecap and behind the knee. The number of magnets or patches will vary with the circumference of your limbs. Leave them on for 30 minutes twice daily. You might sew small magnets into clothes for convenience. That way, the stimulation can continue as you work and go through the day. The required treatment time and results will vary. Make sure to leave the stimulation in place when you exercise in order to reduce stress pain.

Lymphatic Treatments for Face and Breasts

The body's lymphatic system holds a secret to our health and serenity. Many health professionals believe that the lymph system is one of the ways the body cleanses and balances itself. Gentle and deeply cleansing lymphatic massage is highly recommended for breast comfort and beauty. It often releases emotions that have remained trapped for a lifetime. Massaging the breast and nipples tones internal organs because they are related, in the Chinese meridian system, to the uterus. A nurse once told me that massaging the nipples or nursing your baby after childbirth lifts and tones the uterus to its natural shape because hormones are released.

Dr. Marcie Shapiro, who is in private practice near Berkeley, recommends a warm herbal bath with yarrow to encourage lymph cleansing for the entire body after the monthly menstrual period is finished. At some beauty salons, lymphatic drainage is done in preparation for a seaweed wrap. It may help to relax the body and allow the healing benefits of the seaweed to penetrate deeply.

At home, I recommend this simple method for daily breast lymphatic massage: dip a face cloth into hot water to which you have added 10 drops of pure essential lavender oil. Wash each breast with a circular motion for 50 circles around the nipple, first one direction and then the other (for example, clockwise then counterclockwise.) Lavender is very stimulating because its fresh aroma eases the heart and the emotions. For a refined medical body massage, consult an expert such as Natalie Naigles, who has studied the Hauschka method of healing based on the theories of Dr. Rudolph Steiner.

A Harmonizing Massage

Natalie Naigles at Saratoga Skin Care Center revolutionized my approach to massage and energy healing. Chinese Tuina massage tends to be hard, painful, deep, and bruising. The idea is to beat up the qi (energy) so that it is uncomfortable being stuck in one place. You leave the table limping and grunting as your circulation finds new and better paths to follow.

Natalie's gentle "Harmonizing Massage" based on Rudolph Steiner's theories about energetics and Dr. Hauschka's and Weleda's fine European skin care products works deeply because it uses the etheric body—the energy body—that we stimulate in acupuncture. Natalie is lovely, gentle, and mothering. Her movements are slow, meditative, and always lead toward the heart so that impurities can be gathered and released by the kidneys. After a massage with her, I got off the table feeling warm, calm, and centered. Then in about two hours, the skin over my entire body turned bright pink and felt slightly warm. That continued for an hour and then I gradually cooled to normal. My lymph toxins were gone with the wind. Some people may experience less physical and more psychological cleansing effects from the same sort of treatment. The treatment varies with individual needs. Here is a summary of the warming massage Natalie gave me. The strokes are always gentle and lead toward the heart or kidneys to increase cleansing.

- Foot soak with water and (warming) sage oil
- Massage with Dr. Hauschka Rosemary Foot Balm and St. John's Wort Foot Cream (a.k.a. Happy Feet)
- Massage on back and legs with Dr. Hauschka's rose oil (relaxing)

Natalie sometimes made a double-loop infinity sign as a massage motion. Massage oils are chosen according to your temperament—phlegmatic, sanguine, choleric, or melancholic.

Natural Elixir Beverages

Natalie's lymphatic massage also includes one or more Hauschka liquid elixirs, which are used to increase the action of the massage. Depending on your energetic type, they are normally taken as 10–20 drops in water as a beverage.

- Rose (cooling) is harmonizing for a calming effect or for difficult digestion. Red rose buds are used as a tea for angry depression, liver problems, and allergies.
- Elder flower (warming) is "warming, softens hardening, activates sweating, and resolves mucus congestion." Elder brings impurities to the surface to be expelled through the skin.
- Quince is laxative. It moistens the colon, lungs, and skin.
- Blackthorn cleanses the digestive system, tones metabolism, and stimulates creative processes. It is an ideal spring cleansing tonic.

Natalie says that most of her clients lose 10–15 pounds of water weight from a series of 10 treatments. I can think of no more enjoyable way to purify and slim the body. A sensitive practitioner and pleasing atmosphere are very important. I do not recommend having lymphatic massage in a beauty salon, where chemical odors can be asphyxiating. If your massage professional smokes, unloads their personal problems, or preaches while they work, you should leave.

A Lymphatic Anti-Wrinkle Treatment

Based on Natalie's advice, you can tone your facial connective tissue and reduce wrinkles daily. Stand over a bowl containing one cup of very hot water, and add 10 drops of Dr. Hauschka's Lavender Body Oil. Its spicy fragrance combines lavender, moss, horsetail, horse chestnut, geranium, rosemary, and olive oil. Dip a clean, white cotton facecloth into the water, squeeze and apply it damp to your face so that you inhale the steam. Then press downward from the forehead over your entire face, with eyes closed, and over your neck toward your heart. Your skin will be flushed with bright color as you strengthen the lymph system.

Apply a little extra Lavender Body Oil to your wrinkles. Warm a teaspoon under a hot water faucet. Gently "iron" your wrinkles with the back of the spoon. Move downward and inward toward the nose and mouth on the face. Apply extra pressure at the temples and around the mouth. Press downward on the neck toward the heart.

Lavender, according to Dr. Steiner, protects us from "radiation and cosmic pollution." Dab essential oil of lavender on your forehead, neck, shoulders, and heart and let the fragrance open your senses.

Homeopathic Gold for Heart and Mind

An old Chinese doctor once advised, "When many things are wrong with a person, when they have many symptoms and are not getting better from treatments, treat the heart to heal the spirit." The spirit in the heart progresses healing. A happy heart also improves beauty. Steiner also aimed to enhance our inner harmony and realign us with the benevolent universe. Steiner studied eastern and western mysticism, probably the Kabbalah, and matched plants and metals to stimulate corresponding organs. For example, gold (warming) stimulates the heart, and copper (cooling) the kidneys. A homeopath once told me that homeopathic gold, depending on the symptoms, can be recommended for prevention of breast cancer, a disease intimately related to mood, emotions, and circulation.

Homeopathic gold (aurum metallicum) is used most often for severe depression because it regulates heart energy. Is your life stuck in a bad place?

Homeopathic gold is especially suited for oversensitive, despondent people often with high blood pressure, constipation, liver or rib pain, swollen belly or ascites, self-blame, or disgust for life. Also irregular heart beat, dyspnea at night, sores in the nose, and double vision. Check with your homeopathic specialist to determine whether or not to use this remedy and what strength to use.

Happy Garden Tea

The label of Happy Garden Tea reads: "Yin/Yang Sisters invites you into your own secret garden with a delicious flower tea. Dates, licorice, roses, and gardenia welcome you to quiet contentment. People who are upset or women with menopausal discomforts are turning more and more to pleasant-tasting natural teas. It is wise to increase liquid intake during times of stress in order to help the body and mind to regain balance. Happy Garden Tea is a safe, time-honored way to calm worries and cares. Enjoy it warm or chilled."

The ingredients in this instant beverage are bupleurum, mimosa flower, wild jujube date, tender wheat sprout, licorice root, roses, and gardenia buds. Bupleurum (chai hu) is used to help free circulation in the sides and chest. It facilitates liver and gallbladder function and detoxification. Jujube is use to increase energy, and tender wheat sprouts (mai men dong) are moistening for eliminating thirst, dryness, and excess anxiety. Roses and gardenia buds help move stuck circulation and reduce mucus congestion that clouds the senses. Anytime you feel anxious or depressed, sit quietly, take a few deep breaths, and enjoy a comforting warm cup of Happy Garden Tea. Nature's beautiful garden is inside you.

Pain Makes You Squint

Low energy and poor circulation lead to chronic pain and wrinkles, the downside of growing older. An invigorating herbal beverage sends blood and oxygen to where they are needed to smooth, nourish, and rejuvenate the skin, muscles, and joints. Improving energy is always the first step in improving beauty. If your energy sags, your face sags. The following two teas keep energy and endurance high to prevent a tired face and body.

Romantic High

Romantic High is a Yin/Yang Sisters instant beverage that, as the label says, works best for "men and women who want more from romance than books and movies can offer." Romantic High reduces fatigue and backache while it improves loving energy. That in turn improves circulation and mood. Used regularly, "it may light the fires of passion with safe herbs long recommended as sexual tonics." The label warns not to use this tea during colds, head-ache, or fever. It is warming and stimulating and can therefore raise your temperature.

Several of its ingredients, such as morinda, curculigo, and epimedium, increase natural testosterone. Ligustrum, dodder seed, astragalus, cistanches, myrrh, and eucommia bark reduce fatigue and backache. This warm tea can enhance a beautifying glow of contentment for the skin and ease chronic aches from cold weather, overwork, and stress.

Romantic High instant beverage can be enjoyed anytime as a delicious energizing tea. I recommend 1–2 packets daily, as needed, for a naturally satisfying lift.

Gorgeous You

A clear glowing complexion free of blemishes and wrinkles is the natural result of good health. Gorgeous You Instant Beverage from Yin/Yang Sisters contains deep cleansing and immune-enhancing herbs combined with herbs that increase circulation in order to promote good looks and sex appeal. It is wise to increase your liquid intake as part of a general health and beauty program. Gorgeous You is a satisfying way to do this. It can be enjoyed any time of day as part of a natural beauty program designed to keep you radiant, young, and strong.

The ingredients are astragalus, poria, atractylodes, salvia, chinaberry fruit, reishi mushroom, curcuma root, oldenlandia, artemisia, and gardenia bud. The recommended dose is 1–3 packets daily between meals.

Salvia and curcuma (turmeric root) free circulation. Oldenlandia, artemisia, and gardenia buds deep cleanse impurities that can trouble the complexion. Poria and atractylodes are digestive herbs that help to reduce water retention and clarify the senses. Reishi (ling zhi) mushroom and astragalus bring renewed vitality and glow to complexion. Gorgeous You Instant Beverage is recommended as a beautifying tea for men or women who want to deep cleanse, strengthen vitality, and "look and feel gorgeous at any age!"

Is DHEA for You?

Dehydroepiandrosterone (DHEA) is a steroid hormone made by the adrenal glands. It is involved in the production of other hormones such as estrogen, testosterone, and cortisone. It is said to increase metabolism and immune functions and reduce stress. An expensive DHEA wrinkle cream has been touted as a beauty treatment. Some say that you would have to use quite a lot to have any effects, and that the effects stop with disuse. It sounds like a drug dependence with certain pluses and minuses. According to Dr. Yves Requena, an endocrinologist who practices Chinese medicine in France, DHEA is naturally synthesized in the body from a combination of vitamin E and Chinese white yam (*Dioscorea hypoglauca,* in Chinese *bei xie* or *shan yao*).

I personally resist hormone replacement treatments. You can stimulate hormones with herbs such as Siberian ginseng or epimedium for testosterone as long as you use a comfortable dose and combine them with moistening herbs such as American ginseng and lycium fruit. For the rejuvenating, anti-stress effects of estrogen, I prefer Chinese blood-enhancing herbs such as a daily tea made with one handful each of rehmannia glutinosa (shu di huang) and cistanches (rou cong rong) simmered in one quart of water for half an hour.

Another great rejuvenating combination of East Indian herbs is ¼ teaspoon or 1 capsule of ashwagandha along with 1 capsule of shilajet two or three times daily. Ashwagandha strengthens muscle tone and energy like a source of testosterone without irritating side effects. Shilajet, made from coal bitumen, is moistening, stress reducing, and rejuvenating for blood, bones, skin, hair, sexuality, and nerves. If you are too hot and dry, use only Shilajet. If you are sexually weak and chilled or suffer from muscle weakness, numbness, or paralysis, use more ashwagandha.

A Quick Fix for Renewed Youth and Beauty

In *Personal Renewal,* I described ways to take a beautifying vacation at home with virtual trips to the beach or your favorite getaway spot. This time, let's give a party. Invite friends you would like to hug and chat with.

Serve Gorgeous You or Happy Garden Tea. Sit comfortably and massage each other's feet. Chat about your feelings for each other. Do the very balancing hormonal massage found in *Personal Renewal* to feel close, happy, and safe.

Treat yourself regularly to a natural facelift. Among New York acupuncturists, few specialize in acu-beauty treatments. I recommend Dar Godal at his Chelsea Acupuncture clinic on West 23rd Street in Manhattan. His complete facelift program includes needle acupuncture, herbal supplements, and a special salve for home use. His caring manner and dedication are commendable and his results are good.

Especially for Men

Getting out of shape makes men feel old. Lack of exercise also increases the risk of heart trouble, diabetes, and uglifying problems. Prostate health can be improved with a wise, high-alkaline diet including leafy greens, broccoli, and fresh fruits; daily diuretic herbs such as kai kit pills and dandelion, cilantro, and parsley added to salad or made into tea; and plenty of exercise.

Dance your cares and pounds away. We would love to go dancing with you. It is so romantic. Dancing is good for your heart in many ways.

Lola's Way

Spa vacations are a relaxing way to rejuvenate with a loved one. One spa within reach of Washington, D.C., and a former refuge for young George Washington, is located just across the Pennsylvania border in Berkeley Springs, West Virginia. Indians and settlers frolicked, drank, and bathed in the bubbly sulphurated water. Today, a modern, state-run spa includes Roman baths, steam cabinets, and olive oil massage treatments.

George Washington, a young relation and protege of wealthy Lord Fairfax, was a surveyor who grabbed most of what would become Ohio. Periodically, he visited Berkeley Springs to take the waters and diddle the chamber maids. However, he was neither a picture of health nor beauty. George wore terrible wooden false teeth, probably because of his rich diet.

Berkeley Springs is a good place to relax and cleanse. I like to fast on apples and celery, drink the bubbly water, and take homeopathic remedies. Homeopathy Works, a manufacturer and distributer of homeopathic products for people and pets, is across the street from the Roman baths. The wry manner of owner Joe Lillard reminds me of Mark Twain. After a private consultation with one of the town's homeopathic practitioners, you can add your remedies to the water. I often combine homeopathic kali. mur 6x (potassium) and natrum sulphate 6x (sodium) to cleanse both body and mind. The first one ignites the fire of metabolism; the second clears impure fluids. Both rejuvenating minerals help you feel light and clear.

A Healing Ritual

My mother, whether driving though town or country, often scatters wildflower seeds. A green thumb is hereditary in our family. You may wish to spread seeds of beauty in other ways. Its full expression requires tranquility and vision. Natural beauty is the magic with which we recreate ourselves. Our appearance, thoughts, and actions shape us as much as our relationships and surroundings.

Feng Shui, an ancient Chinese art, seeks to harmonize the individual with his or her environment. Recently, it has taken on a practical application by interior decorators, who choose colors, shapes, and sounds to create an attractive and healthful setting. However, the original form is mystical. The practice invokes the fire of creativity and the water of inspiration. It invites Spirit inside. Feng Shui has a lot in common with Western magic because both seek blessings and protection from evil influences with ritual. In a prayer to the Greek god Helios found in the *Papyrus Mimaut* at the Louvre museum, we find this invocation: "Come to me with a happy face, giving me sustenance, health, safety, wealth, the blessing of children, knowledge, a good name (fame), goodwill from others, sound judgement, honor, memory, grace, shapeliness, beauty in the eyes of all men who see me—you, who hear me in everything whatsoever, hear my prayers."

Our ritual, based on internal feng shui, will help you to look into the future. Sit quietly and imagine yourself inside a large crystal ball. Mentally observe:

Ahead of you is your future.
To the right are love and family.
To the left are power, wealth, and education.
Behind you are career and helpful friends.
Where do you need to add more light and beauty?

This book is an invitation to enhance your vitality and natural gifts, which will enlarge your relationship with Beauty and Spirit in all aspects of life. Beauty begins inside us and reaches far beyond our understanding. It is a journey that never ends.

Annotated Resource Guide

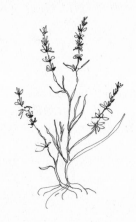

Designer Oscar de la Renta has said, "Beauty is a state of mind." Using environmentally friendly ingredients improves your looks and your sleep. It takes a load off your conscience. You can trust ingredients that are good enough to eat. Quite a number of cosmetic companies make it their business to use natural, vegetarian ingredients and cruelty-free testing methods. The listings in each section begin with my personal favorites and also contain general company information. The sections cover products and services from:

- Health-food stores, supermarkets, and bargain outlets
- Specialty shops or famous-name beauty salons
- Stores and internet sources carrying Asian herbs and remedies
- Homeopathic products manufacturers and distributors
- Foreign listings for natural beauty products
- Health and beauty professionals

Because of space limitations, this resource guide is far from complete. However, it offers inspiring examples of health-minded people who have created top quality, environmentally sound beauty products and highly successful companies. Their growing influence is felt everywhere.

HEALTH-FOOD STORES, SUPERMARKETS, AND OUTLETS

Natural Beauty Products for External Use

The following products are easily found in American health-food stores. You can look for them in CVS, Rite Aid, Wal-Mart, and your local supermarket. Their reasonable prices and excellent quality are well worth it.

Kiss My Face Inc.
144 Main Street
Gardiner, NY 12525
Phone: 845-255-0884
www.kissmyface.com

Kiss My Face Corporation, located in a converted barn and feed store in Gardiner, New York, was started by two handsome vegans living on a 200-acre organic farm in the Hudson River Valley. Bob McCloud has a business degree and Stephen Byckiewicz is a painter whose work is currently showing in a Miami Beach gallery.

One evening in the 1980s, in front of a crackling fire in their old farmhouse, they made a lifelong pact to take on the modern cosmetic industry by making natural, vegetarian, cruelty-free (non-animal tested) beauty products. They loaded their first item, big bars of green-colored olive oil soap, along with lots of organic vegetables into the back of their yellow Volkswagen bug and drove to New York in search of financial backing. By the time the vegetables ran out, they had found backers.

Since then, their company has created over 150 beauty products that combine vitamins, minerals, botanicals, and essential oils without chemical additives, artificial fragrances, synthetic colors, or animal testing. Several of their body oils and their facial Botanical Acne Gel contain ingredients safe enough to eat. In this book, look for Kiss My Face products in chapters dealing with beautiful complexion, home facials, healthy makeup, and hair and scalp treatments.

Kiss My Face contributes to AIDS organizations, environmentally minded groups (including the Nature Conservancy), and the Southern Poverty Law Center.

Jason Natural Cosmetics
Culver City, CA 90232-2484
Phone: 310-838-7543 or 1-800-527-6605
www.jasonproducts.com

Jason Natural Cosmetics Company, located in Culver City, California, makes health-food store products for the hair, skin, body, and teeth. A skip and a hop from Hollywood, they began as a cosmetic company that serviced salons and movie studios. After they were taken over in 1959 by a new president, Jeffry B. Light, who was previously associated with Haines foods, the company took a strong environmentally friendly turn.

At Jason, vegetarian philosophy is strictly observed: their aromatherapy, phytotherapy, herbology, vitamins and minerals, organic botanicals, and high-quality food-grade nutraceutical ingredients contain no animal ingredients and have minimal chemicals and preservatives. The company gives a generous share of its profits to many environmental causes.

Weleda Inc.
Congers, NY 10920
Phone: 1-877-293-5332
www.weleda.com

Weleda was created in 1921 in Switzerland by physician and mystic Dr. Rudolph Steiner, who was dedicated to the study of "relationships between the substances and processes of nature and the human being." The name Weleda refers to an ancient tradition of Celtic women healers. I especially like their extra mild shampoos (for children and adults) that boost natural highlights.

I apply Weleda's essential rosemary oil to my face and scalp before taking a sauna. Heat and massage make the oil penetrate for a fragrant and gently exfoliating oil treatment.

Aveda
140 Fifth Avenue
New York, NY 10011
Phone: 1-800-AVEDA-24
www.aveda.com

Aveda, one of 17 brands formed by the Estee Lauder family, makes an "all sensitive line" that contains a shampoo and conditioner that was tested at John Hopkins University and found to be 99.9% effective in causing no irritation. It contains no alcohol, coloring, or fragrance. The water-based shampoo and conditioner contain geranium to cleanse excess oil and dirt. Aveda, known for its flower-essence-based products, also makes after-shampoo hair conditioners such as Sap Moss conditioner, which restores moisture for dry damaged hair, and Curessence, a protein conditioner that seals split ends and coats the hair shaft to protect it.

Burt's Bees, Inc.
Raleigh, NC 27675
Phone: 1-800-849-7112
www.burtsbees.com

Burt's Bees started in a trailer in the 1990s. Burt Shavitz, the cute, hippie-looking, gray haired, bearded man sitting on a motorcycle in the company poster, left New York for Maine to get away from it all (including money). He became known as the town's eccentric vegetarian beekeeper. His friend, Roxanne Quimby, used her chemistry background to make great things like candles and salves using Burt's leftover beeswax. The company, now located in Durham, North Carolina, makes over 100 healthy beauty products that contain plant extracts, vitamins, food flavors, and, of course, beeswax.

Health Foods

California

Bernard Jensen International
1914 West Mission Road, Suite F
Escondido, CA 92029
Phone: 760-291-1255
E-mail: info@bernardjensenintl.com
(Dr. Bernard Jensen's books, videos, and nutritional products)

New York

Integral Yoga Natural Foods
234 West 13th Street
New York, NY 10011
Phone: 212-243-2642
www.iynaturalfoods.com

A Matter of Health
1478 First Avenue (at 77th Street)
New York, NY 10021
Phone: 212-288-8280

SPECIALTY SHOPS AND BEAUTY SALONS

Georgette Klinger
Phone:1-800-KLINGER
www.GeorgetteKlinger.com

Georgette Klinger's eight salon locations—in New York; Short Hills, New Jersey; Beverly Hills; Costa Mesa, California; Dallas; Washington, D.C.; Chicago; and Palm Beach, Florida—offer individualized skin care analysis and facials, scalp and hair treatments, therapeutic body massage, exfoliating herbal and seaweed body treatments, facial dermabrasion, makeup services, hair styling, manicures, pedicures, and waxing.

Georgette Klinger offers an extensive collection of exclusive at-home products formulated to meet individual skincare needs. The salons also feature special seasonal offers, corporate programs, and youth facial treatments. For your convenience, the website has a Q & A section.

Origins
Phone: 1-800-ORIGINS
www.origins.com

Origins, Estee Lauder's flagship natural products company, began 10 years ago by making lifestyle products designed to "bring men and women of all ages a sense of harmony, health and happiness. Inside and out." Their brochures read like new age doctrine, and their health-minded products have attractive packaging that make them suitable for gifts. Try Origins Herbal Salt Scrubs, Skin Souffles, Body Gloss, and Foot Care products.

Origins specialty shops around the country feature personalized skin care advice and products designed to pamper different skin types. I love the cheerful, real grapefruit aroma of Origins Gloomaway Body Gloss. I spritz it everywhere, even in my hair. It contains jojoba and bitter almond oils, grapefruit, orange, mint, essential oil of cinnamon, and camphor. It tantalizes your senses and opens your breathing. Pomegranate Polish Salt Scrub, Origins latest product, uses tangy pomegranate seed extract as a natural exfoliator.

Avon Products, Inc.
New York, NY 10020
Phone: 1-800-FOR-AVON
www.avon.com

Avon Center Spa at Trump Tower (New York)
Phone: 212-755-2866

Avon, the world's most international beauty company, began 115 years ago. Currently over 3.5 million representatives in 139 countries knock on doors to sell Avon products. Many of them also have websites. I remember with affection the Avon lady of my youth. She was a single mother who might not otherwise have had time to work. For over 50 years, Avon Products Foundation, Inc., has supported a wide range of organizations and programs that foster women's leadership in the United States and around the world.

In 2001, Avon began a wellness line that includes dietary supplements, aromatherapy, and other health-conscious items you can see on their website. Andrea Jung, Avon's (Canadian/Chinese) Chief Executive Officer, has committed to reaching $250 million by the end of 2002 to help achieve their goal to "kiss goodbye to breast cancer."

SUPERSTORES

CVS, ProCare, Rite Aid, Wal-Mart, other discount outlets, and beauty supply companies have a large selection of natural beauty products. Don't hesitate to ask them for skin and hair products such as pearl creams and soaps, natural henna shampoos and conditioners, and vegetable-based semipermanent hair colors originating in Asia, Mexico, and Latin America.

HOMEOPATHIC REMEDIES

You can find homeopathic remedies in most pharmacies and health-food stores. However, there are times when you need to have an individual recommendation or a remedy formulated especially for you.

Homeopathy Works
33 Fairfax Street
Berkeley Springs, WV 25411
Phone: 304-258-2541 or 1-800-336-1695
www.homeopathyworks.com

Homeopathy Works manufactures and sells hundreds of homeopathic products for people and animals. You can subscribe to their friendly informative monthly newsletter from their website.

StatScript Pharmacy
Multiple locations
Phone: 1-866-851-4395
www.chronimed.com

At StatScript Pharmacy's Chelsea store in New York City, Anwar Mahmud, an expert homeopath from Bangladesh, generously recommends remedies for both people and animals. He says, "I want to help everything that lives."

Dolisos Laboratoires
6 rue Brindejonc de Moulinais
31500 Toulouse, France
Phone: 335-62-47-77-00
(Alcohol-based homeopathic products)

ASIAN HERBS AND NATURAL BEAUTY PRODUCTS

California

Wing Hop Fung Ginseng & China Products Center
727 North Broadway
Los Angeles, CA 90012
Phone: 1-800-239-6888
www.winghopfung.com

I met Lan and Keng Ong, owners of the Los Angeles superstore Wing Hop Fung (Cantonese for harmonious, eternal flowering) in 2000. Since then, I have been writing a weekly health newsletter and Q&A column for their website.

Lan and her brother Keng spent their first couple of years in a refugee camp after leaving Vietnam. Their grandfather, a celebrated herbal doctor from China, kept them alive with ginseng. Mom and Dad Ong speak little English, but Lan and Keng are American, cell-phone carrying, college grads who continue the fine family tradition.

Wing Hop Fung sells everything from Chinese clothes, martial arts equipment, housewares and furnishings, and fine art and collectibles to Chinese teas, raw herbs, and many inexpensive Chinese patent remedies (pills and extracts). The store sells Bird's Nest Extract and an attractive satin beauty bag, which contains pearl cream, powdered pearl, and several instant beverages for enhancing the complexion.

East Earth Trade Winds
P.O. Box 493151
Redding, CA 96049-3151
Phone: 1-800-258-6878
www.eastearthtrade.com

I once e-mailed this company's founder, Michel Czehatowski, for his advice on energy tonic herbs for an article I was writing. I received an answer from China, where he was studying advanced acupuncture techniques. His company responds quickly and efficiently. Their catalogue carries Long Hay Flat brand liquid herbal extracts such as Reishi+ and Gentle Rejuvenator. They sell Yin/Yang Sisters Instant Beverages and essential oils that I recommended in several chapters.

East Earth Trade Winds carries carry Chinese bulk herbs, over 350 concentrated herbal extracts from Sanjiu, and many popular Chinese-made patent remedies I mentioned in this book.

Health Concerns
Oakland, California
Phone: 1-800-233-9355

Health Concerns manufactures professional herbal products respected by acupuncturists, herbalists, and physicians. I have recommended a number of their fine products in this book. To order them, you have to consult with a specialist. You can contact me at lethah@earthlink.net, and I can recommend the appropriate herbal pills according to your individual needs and fully explain their use. Ordering requires a password.

Health Concerns has a clinic in Oakland, California, and most of their products are formulated by their Asian herbalist, who is more than 80 years old and thriving. Andrew Gaeddert, the herbalist who founded the company, has written books on Chinese herbs, including *Chinese Herbs in the Western Clinic.*

Intelligent Choice, Inc.
949 South Hope Street, Suite 3140
Los Angeles, CA 90015
Phone: 1-888-252-7873
www.absolutelyhealthy.com

This company specializes in quality Japanese nutritional supplements made with foods that naturally enhance beauty. Asitaba is a root that clears the complexion as it reduces cholesterol and protects vitality. Konjac is a weight-loss pill made from konnyaku, a yam that reduces fat and cholesterol. See their website for research information on LEM, a concentrated form of shiitake mushroom sold in capsules by Intelligent Choice.

Nha Thuoc Van Hoi Xuan
Chinese Herbs & Ginseng Inc.
9200 Bolsa Avenue #102
Westminster, CA 92683
Phone: 714-893-2922
Fax: 714-893-0140

Little Saigon, located 40 minutes from Los Angeles in Westminster, has a wide selection of malls with vast shopping centers, beauty shops, and clothing stores specializing in attractive Chinese and Vietnamese items. Everyone speaks English. Beauty shops in the huge mall at 9200 Bolsa offer facials, dermabrasion, and nonsurgical facelifts.

New York

Lin Sisters Herb Shop
4 Bowery Street
New York, NY 10003
Phone: 212-962-5417
Fax: 212-587-8826
E-mail: linsisterherbs@aol.com

Susan Sha and her brother Frank have been, it seems, life long friends from New York's Chinatown. I chose Susan to appear in my *Asian Health Secrets* home video (available from Amazon.com), which shares health and beauty secrets of our Chinese neighbors. Susan is cheery and attractive, a fine traditional Chinese herbalist with a sympathetic ear for her American customers. Her beauty potions include specially formulated herbal soups and powders for age spots and wrinkles.

Lin Sisters herb shop sells Yin/Yang Sisters instant beverages, which Susan designed along with one of the largest and best herbal medicine companies in China.

Foods of India
121 Lexington Avenue
New York, NY 10016
Phone: 212-683-4419

This store carries all major brands of ayurvedic herbs and natural remedies as well as a large selection of foods. It has the friendliest staff in Manhattan's Little India.

Butala Emporium Inc.
108 East 28 Street
New York, NY 10016
Phone: 212-684-4447
Email: service@indousbooks.com
www.indousplaza.com

This company, with locations in New York and New Jersey, specializes in Ayurvedic medicines, beauty products, and books.

Texas

Himalaya USA
6950 Portwest Drive, Suite 170
Houston, TX 77024
Phone: 713-863-1686 or 1-800-869-4640
www.himalayausa.com
(Dermacare skin supplements and nail care capsules in Whole Foods and Wild Oats)

Washington State

Fungi Perfecti (Medicinal Mushrooms Specialist)
P.O. Box 7634
Olympia, WA 98507
Phone: 1-800-780-9126
www.fungi.com

FOREIGN SOURCES

Canada

La Beaute Dans La Nature
49 Dufferin Road
Hampstead, PQ H3X2X7
Phone: 514-489-2344
Fax: 514-488-6113
(Healthy cosmetics and beauty supplies)

Medicinal Plant Products Inc
250 6th Avenue SW, Suite 940
Calgary, AB T2P3H7
Phone: 403-261-8888
Fax: 403-264-3310

France

5 Saisons Elixirs Energetiques
Propos' Nature SARL
BP 53-13840 Rognes, France
Phone: 04-42-50-30-40
Fax: 04-42-50-34-38
www.5saisons.com

Journalist Marie Borrel has written *Le Guide des Elixirs Energetiques* (Guy Tredaniel, Paris, 2001) to explain how these herbal extracts work and how to use them. They are Western herbs formulated to balance the Chinese Five Elements. The elixirs are based on the writings of Dr. Yves Requena (mentioned in my list of favorites at the end of this chapter).

Nickel
Spa for Men
www.nickel.fr
(Men's facial products)

Germany

Herba Natura
HERBA.NATURA@t-online.de

The largest wholesaler of Chinese herbs in Germany, which sells over 300 Chinese raw herbs. Owner Harold Noll makes regular trips to China to check that production runs according to GMP standards. The company sells Chinese patent formulas and acupuncture supplies.

Israel

Galilee Herbal Remedies
Kfar Hannasi
Upper Galilee 12305, Israel
Phone: 972-6-6914833
Fax: 972-6-6914726

Mexico

Grisi HNOS, S.A. de C.V
Toiletries Division
Amores # 1746
03100 Mexico D.F.
(Madre Perla crema—mother of pearl cream)

MY FAVORITE HEALTH AND BEAUTY PROFESSIONALS

California

Marietta Carter-Narcisse
1438-½ South Robertson Boulevard, Suite 1
Los Angeles, CA 90035-3411
Phone: 310-205-9185
E-mail: info@mariettacarternarcisse.com
(Makeup for film, workshops, Calypso Cosmetics)

New York

Gad Cohen
New York, NY
Phone: 212-366-0302
www.gadcohen.com
(Expert stylist for makeup and haircut and color)

Clif deRaita at Georgette Klinger
501 Madison Avenue
New York, NY
Phone: 212-838-3200 ext. 328
(Expert makeup and style instruction)

Sakura Beauty
17 East Broadway, Room 206
New York, NY 10002
Phone: 212-393-1144
(Micro-dermabrasion)

Shangri-La Day Spa
247 West 72 Street
New York, NY 10022
Phone: 212-579-0615

A Tibetan-run beauty salon with a monastery atmosphere, they specialize in facials using Rene Guinot products from France and Tibetan herbal detox and relaxation massage and wraps. Their Sorig Therapeutic massage oil is made from Tibetan herbs and sunflower oil in Dharamsala, India.

Virginia Fry
Avon Centre at Trump Tower
725 Fifth Avenue
New York, NY 10022
Phone: 212-755-AVON
www.avon.com

Susan Lin, (See Lin Sisters Herb Shop)

Dr. Lili Wu See Lin Sisters
420 West 24 Street, 1D
New York, NY 10011
Phone: 212-741-6674

Lili is an expert Shanghai-trained acupuncturist and traditional Chinese herbalist who treats a variety of health and beauty issues with great success and kindness. She also has a Brooklyn location (Phone: 718-439-8805).

Ildar Gadol
Chelsea Healing
216 West 23rd Street
New York, NY 10011
Phone: 212-645-6447
www.chelseahealing.com
(Acupuncture facelifts)

Linda van Horn
Phone: 718-346-2212

Linda's gentle, healing touch combines Japanese Shiatsu and energy balancing. She teaches yoga and healthy lifestyle practices, makes house calls, and takes female clients only.

Natalie Naigles
Saratoga Skin Center
Arcade Building
376 Broadway
Saratoga Springs, NY 12866
Phone: 518-580-8888
(Facials, slimming and rejuvenating lymphatic massage, and quality skin care products)

France

Dr. Yves Requena
13, avenue Victor Hugo
Aix-en-provence 13100, France
Phone: 04-42-26-91-38
Fax: 04-42-26-50-04

Yves is a brilliant western-trained endocrinologist, TCM acupuncturist, herbalist, author of numerous books and video tapes, and director of Institut Europeen de Qi Gong. The address is:

Institut Europeen de Qi Gong
Bastide des Micocoulier
Chateau de Galice
1940, route de Loqui
Aix-en-Provence 13090, France
Phone: 04-42-20-40-85
Fax: 04-42-20-06-58

Index

malabsorption, 150
malaria, 121, 221
manganese deficiency, 137
Mars, Brigitte, 111
Mary Kay, 169
massage, 163, 230–31
mastitis, 227
meals, size of, 43–44
meat eating, adverse effects, 69
memory, 82, 124
men
  abdominal bloating, 220
  damiana, effect of, 33–34
  effects of lack of exercise, 235
  eyes, 143
  flirting, 22–23
  foot care, 115
  groin pain, 220
  herbal sexual tonic, 64
  hair care, 133
  indigestion, 220
  jock itch, 167–68
  skin care for, 154–55, 182
  slimming, 78–79
  soothing inflammation, 101
  style points for, 194
  tension, 220
  testosterone herbs, 88
  voice suggestions for, 208
meningitis, 221
Menken, Adah Isaacs, 172
menopause, 130, 167, 217, 220
menstruation, 99, 100
mental focus, 123, 214, 215
metabolism, speeding, 83
migraines, 50
Miller-Huey, Rita, 67
Mills, Simon, 33
Mindell, Earl, 120
minerals, for hair, 120–21
Mingmu Di Huang Wan, 138
Mobility 2, 63
moisturizing, 46
  herbs, 138
  teas and beverages, 46
moles, 157–59
Monroe, Marilyn, 194–95
Montez, Lola (Eliza Gilbert), 3, 20–22, 79, 88, 104, 132
  bonnets recommended, 36
  defeating stress, 34
  facial treatment, 172–73
  on hair, 119, 133
  hand treatments, 113–14

  hands, language of, 115–16
  opposition to makeup, 182
  on skin, 146
  vocal study, 206
  on walk, 64
moodiness, 68
movement, rejuvenating, 226
MSM, 61, 108, 109
mumps, 218
muscles, 38–40, 80–81
mushrooms, medicinal, 40, 45, 47–48, 50
  beauty and, 28–30
  cooking with, 30
  hot climate and inflammatory symptoms, 42–43
Mycomedicinals: An Informational Booklet on Medicinal Mushrooms (Stamets), 27–28

Naigles, Natalie, 114, 230–31
nails, 110–11
Narcissism, Healthy, 15
Narcissus, 14–15
National Institutes of Health, 137
natural killer cells, 27
nausea, 106
neck tension, 138
Nemesis, 15
nerve growth regeneration, 45
nerves, 38–40
nerve stabilizer, 124
nerve tonics, 27
nervines, 27
nervous disorders, 125
nervous exhaustion, 129
nervous hunger, 76
nervousness, 4, 26, 130, 208, 224
nervous tension, quick fix for, 114–15
nettle, 26, 39, 54, 71, 110, 112, 124, 126–27, 150
neutral ginseng, 62, 83, 184
New York Hospital dermatology clinic, 159
Niccoli, Julian, 36
night sweats, 46, 130, 207
Nine Flavor Tea pills, 96–97, 130
nose, sores in, 233
nux vomica, 50, 68, 91, 224

odors, 40–43
oily skin, care for, 180
Oldenlandia diffusa, 75, 149
Omega 3 and 6 oils, 50, 67, 95
Ong, Lan, 154
On Medical Matters (Dioscorides), 100
oozing wounds, 216
oral sores, 130
Ornish, Dean, 68